Case Files™
Anatomy

Second Edition

EUGENE C. TOY, MD
The John S. Dunn, Senior Academic Chief and Program Director
The Methodist Hospital-Houston
Obstetrics and Gynecology Residency Program
Houston, Texas
Clerkship Director, Clinical Associate Professor
Department of Obstetrics and Gynecology
University of Texas Medical School at Houston
Houston, Texas

LAWRENCE M. ROSS, MD, PHD
Adjunct Professor
Department of Neurobiology and Anatomy
University of Texas Medical School at Houston
Houston, Texas

LEONARD J. CLEARY, PHD
Senior Lecturer
Department of Neurobiology and Anatomy
Course Director, Gross Anatomy
University of Texas Medical School at Houston
Houston, Texas

CRISTO PAPASAKELARIOU, MD, FACOG
Clinical Professor,
Department of Obstetrics and Gynecology
University of Texas Medical Branch
Galveston, Texas
Clinical Director of Gynecologic Surgery
St. Joseph Medical Center
Houston, Texas

McGraw Hill **Medical**

New York   Chicago   San Francisco
Lisbon   London   Madrid   Mexico City
Milan   New Delhi   San Juan   Seoul
Singapore   Sydney   Toronto

Case Files™: Anatomy, Second Edition

1 2 3 4 5 6 7 8 9 0   DOC/DOC   0 9 8

ISBN 978-0-07-148980-5
MHID 0-07-148980-0

Notice

Medicine is an ever-changing science. As new research and clinical experience broaden our knowledge, changes in treatment and drug therapy are required. The authors and the publisher of this work have checked with sources believed to be reliable in their efforts to provide information that is complete and generally in accord with the standard accepted at the time of publication. However, in view of the possibility of human error or changes in medical sciences, neither the editors nor the publisher nor any other party who has been involved in the preparation or publication of this work warrants that the information contained herein is in every respect accurate or complete, and they disclaim all responsibility for any errors or omissions or for the results obtained from use of the information contained in this work. Readers are encouraged to confirm the information contained herein with other sources. For example and in particular, readers are advised to check the product information sheet included in the package of each drug they plan to administer to be certain that the information contained in this work is accurate and that changes have not been made in the recommended dose or in the contraindications for administration. This recommendation is of particular importance in connection with new or infrequently used drugs.

This book was set in Times Roman by International Typesetting and Composition.
The editor was Catherine A. Johnson.
The production supervisor was Catherine Saggese.
Project management was provided by Gita Raman, International Typesetting and Composition.
The cover designer was Aimee Nordin.
RR Donnelley was printer and binder.

This book is printed on acid-free paper.

Library of Congress Cataloging-in-Publication Data

Case files. Anatomy / Eugene C. Toy ... [et al.].—2nd ed.
    p. ; cm.
    Includes index.
    Rev. ed. of: Case files. Gross anatomy. 2005.
    ISBN-13: 978-0-07-148980-5 (pbk. : alk. paper)
    ISBN-10: 0-07-148980-0 (pbk. alk. paper)
      1. Anatomy, Pathological—Case studies.   I. Toy, Eugene C.   II. Case files.
  Gross anatomy.   III. Title: Anatomy.
      [DNLM: 1. Anatomy—Problems and Exercises.   2. Clinical Medicine—
  Problems and Exercises. QS 18.2 C337 2008]
  RB25.C265 2008
  611—dc22   2007038255

❖ DEDICATION

Hitoshi "Toshi" Nikaidoh (1968–2003)

We dedicate this book to our dear friend, Dr. Toshi Nikaidoh, who led by example, always beyond the call of duty and along the way, taught so many of us about so many important things about life.

As a surgeon-to-be, he tutored fellow lower-level medical students not only how to master the challenges of gross anatomy, but also how to develop the skillful art of dissection and respect for the human body.

As a spiritual leader, he taught his youth group not only the meaning of good fellowship by recalling good times spent on missionary travels abroad, but also the value of good worship by sharing his faith along the way.

As a physician, he taught patients not only to hope when all hope is lost, but also to have faith through which peace can be found.

And as a friend, son, brother, or just that smiling doctor in the hallway with the bow tie, he taught us how truly possible it is for one person to make a world of difference.

Toshi's dedication to academics and education, his compassion for the sick and less fortunate, and his tireless devotion to his faith, family, and friends have all continued to touch and change lives of all who knew him and even of all who only knew of him.

Miki Takase, MD
Fellow classmate,
University of Texas Medical School at Houston
St. Joseph Medical Center Ob/Gyn Resident

Written in behalf of Toshi's many friends,
classmates, fellow residents, staff, and faculty at
University of Texas Medical School at Houston and
St. Joseph Medical Center

In the memory of Dr. Hitoshi Nikaidoh, who demonstrated unselfishness, love for his fellow man, and compassion for everyone around him. He is the best example of the physician healer, and we were blessed to have known him.

—ECT

To my wife, Irene; the children, Chip, Jennifer, Jocelyn, Tricia, and Trey; and the medical students, each of whom has taught me something of value.

—LMR

For the students at the University of Texas Medical School at Houston, with thanks to Dr. John Byrne for his support of the Human Structure Facility.

—LJC

To my parents Kiriaki and Alexander, and my wife Beth, for their support, love, and encouragement.

—CP

❖ CONTENTS

❖ CONTRIBUTORS

John E. Bertini, Jr., MD, FACS
Academic Chief
Department of Urology
St. Joseph Medical Center
Houston, Texas
Benign Prostatic Hypertrophy
Testicular Cancer

Konrad P. Harms, MD
Associate Program Director
Obstetrics and Gynecology Residency Program
The Methodist Hospital-Houston
Houston, Texas
Clinical Assistant Professor
Weill Cornell School of Medicine
New York, New York
Greater Vestibular Gland Abscess

Lauren Giacobbe, MD
Resident in Obstetrics and Gynecology
The Methodist Hospital-Houston
Houston, Texas
Ectopic Pregnancy

Christie S. Keil
Medical Student, Class of 2008
University of Texas Medical School at Houston
Houston, Texas
Carotid Insufficiency
Suprarenal (Adrenal) Tumors

Lindsey Kelly
Medical Student, Class of 2008
University of Texas Medical School at Houston
Houston, Texas
Ectopic Pregnancy
Greater Vestibular Gland

Vian Nguyen, MD
Resident in Obstetrics and Gynecology
The Methodist Hospital-Houston
Houston, Texas
Cephalohematoma
Cervical Cancer

Jeané Simmons Holmes, MD, FACOG
Assistant Clinical Professor
Weill Cornell School of Medicine
New York, New York
Obstetrics and Gynecology Residency Program
The Methodist Hospital-Houston
Houston, Texas
Cervical Cancer

Brad Blachly Swelstad, MD
Chief Resident in Obstetrics and Gynecology
The Methodist Hospital-Houston
Houston, Texas
Injury to Inferior Epigastric Artery

Thomas V. Taylor, MD, FACS, FRCS
Academic Chief of Surgery
St. Joseph Medical Center
Houston, Texas
Acute Appendicitis
Inguinal Hernia

Kathryn A. Winslow, MD
Resident in Obstetrics and Gynecology
The Methodist Hospital-Houston
Houston, Texas
Pulmonary Embolism

❖ ACKNOWLEDGMENTS

The inspiration for this basic science series occurred at an educational retreat led by Dr. Maximillian Buja, who at the time was the Dean of the medical school. Dr. Buja, served as Dean of the University of Texas Medical School at Houston from 1995 to 2003, before being appointed Executive Vice President for Academic Affairs. It has been such a joy to work together with Drs. Len Cleary and Lawrence Ross, who are brilliant anatomists and teachers. Sitting side by side during the writing process as they precisely described the anatomical structures was academically fulfilling, but more so, made me a better surgeon. It has been a privilege to work with Dr. Cristo Papasakelariou, a dear friend, scientist, leader, and the finest gynecological laparoscopic surgeon I know. I would like to thank McGraw-Hill for believing in the concept of teaching by clinical cases. I owe a great debt to Catherine Johnson, who has been a fantastically encouraging and enthusiastic editor. I greatly appreciate the talented, thorough and insightful review by Christie Keil, a fourth year medical student. Drs. Cleary and Ross would like to acknowledge the figure drawings from the University of Texas Medical School at Houston originally published in Philo et al., *Guide to Human Anatomy*. Philadelphia: Saunders, 1985. At Methodist Hospital, I appreciate Drs. Mark Boom, Karin Pollock-Larsen, H. Dirk Sostman, and Judy Paukert, and Mr. John Lyle and Mr. Reggie Abraham. At St. Joseph Medical Center, I would like to recognize our outstanding administrators: Phil Robinson, Pat Mathews, Laura Fortin, Dori Upton, Cecile Reynolds, and Drs. John Bertini and Thomas V. Taylor. I appreciate Marla Buffington's advice and assistance. Without the help from my colleagues, Drs. Sam Law, Eric Haufrect, Keith Reeves, and Waverly Peakes, this manuscript could not have been written. Most importantly, I am humbled by the love, affection, and encouragement from my lovely wife, Terri, and our four children, Andy, Michael, Allison, and Christina.

Eugene C. Toy

❖ INTRODUCTION

Mastering the diverse knowledge within a field such as anatomy is a formidable task. It is even more difficult to draw on that knowledge, relate it to a clinical setting, and apply it to the context of the individual patient. To gain these skills, the student learns best with good anatomical models or a well-dissected cadaver, at the laboratory bench, guided and instructed by experienced teachers, and inspired toward self-directed, diligent reading. Clearly, there is no replacement for education at the bench. Even with accurate knowledge of the basic science, the application of that knowledge is not always easy. Thus, this collection of patient cases is designed to simulate the clinical approach and stress the clinical relevance to the anatomical sciences.

Most importantly, the explanations for the cases emphasize the mechanisms and structure–function principles, rather than merely rote questions and answers. This book is organized for versatility to allow the student "in a rush" to go quickly through the scenarios and check the corresponding answers or to consider the thought-provoking explanations. The answers are arranged from simple to complex: the bare answers, a clinical correlation of the case, an approach to the pertinent topic including objectives and definitions, a comprehension test at the end, anatomical pearls for emphasis, and a list of references for further reading. The clinical vignettes are listed by region to allow for a more synthetic approach to the material. A listing of cases is included in Section III to aid the student who desires to test his/her knowledge of a certain area or to review a topic including basic definitions. We intentionally used open-ended questions in the case scenarios to encourage the student to think through relations and mechanisms.

Applying Basic Sciences to Clinical Situations

APPROACH TO LEARNING

Learning anatomy is not just memorization. It is the visualization of the relations between the various structures of the body and the understanding of their corresponding functions. Rote memorization will lead to quick forgetfulness and boredom. Instead, the student should approach an anatomical structure by trying to correlate its purpose with its design. Structures that are close together should be related not only spatially but also functionally. The student should also try to project clinical significance to the anatomical findings. For example, if two nerves travel close together down the arm, one could speculate that a tumor, laceration, or ischemic injury might affect both nerves; the next step would be to describe the deficits expected on the physical examination.

The student must approach the subject in a systematic manner, by studying the **skeletal** relations of a certain region of the body, **the joints, the muscular system, the cardiovascular system** (including arterial perfusion and venous drainage), **the nervous system** (such as sensory and motor neural innervations), and the **skin**. Each bone or muscle is unique and has advantages due to its structure and limitations or perhaps vulnerability to specific injuries. The student is encouraged to read through the description of the anatomical relation in a certain region, correlate the illustrations of the same structures, and then try to envision the anatomy in three dimensions. For instance, if the anatomical drawings are in the coronal plane, the student may want to draw the same region in the sagittal or cross-sectional plane as an exercise to visualize the anatomy more clearly.

BASIC TERMINOLOGY

Anatomical position: The basis of all descriptions in the anatomical sciences, with the head, eyes, and toes pointing forward, the upper limbs by the side with the palms facing forward, and the lower limbs together.

Anatomical planes: A section through the body, one of four commonly described planes. The **median plane** is a single vertically oriented plane dividing the body into right and left halves, whereas the **sagittal planes** are oriented parallel to the median plane but not necessarily in the midline. **Coronal planes** are perpendicular to the median plane and divide the body into anterior (front) and posterior (back) portions. **Transverse, axial, or cross-sectional planes** pass through the body perpendicular to the median and coronal planes and divide the body into upper and lower parts.

Directionality: Superior (cranial) is toward the head, whereas **inferior (caudal)** is toward the feet; **medial** is toward the midline, whereas **lateral** is away from the midline. **Proximal** is toward the trunk or attachment, whereas **distal** is away from the trunk or attachment. **Superficial** is near the surface, whereas **deep** is away from the surface.

Motion: Adduction is movement toward the midline, whereas **abduction** is movement away from the midline. **Extension** is straightening a part of the body, whereas **flexion** is bending the structure. **Pronation** is the action of rotating the palmar side of the forearm facing posteriorly, whereas **supination** is the action of rotating the palmar side of the forearm anteriorly.

APPROACH TO READING

The student should **read with a purpose** and not merely to memorize facts. Reading with the goal of comprehending the relation between structure and function is one of the keys to anatomy. Also, being able to relate the anatomical sciences to the clinical picture is critical. Thus, there are seven key questions that help to stimulate the application of basic science information to the clinical setting.

1. **Given the importance of a certain required function, which anatomical structure provides the ability to perform that function?**
2. **Given the anatomical description of a body part, what is its function?**
3. **Given a patient's symptoms, what structure is affected?**
4. **Which lymph nodes are most likely to be affected by cancer at a particular location?**
5. **If an injury occurs to one part of the body, what is the expected clinical manifestation?**
6. **Given a deficit such as weakness or numbness, what other symptoms or signs would the patient most likely have?**
7. **What is the male or female homologue to the organ in question?**

1. **Given the importance of a certain required function, which anatomical structure provides the ability to perform that function?**
    The student should be able to relate the anatomical structure to a function. When approaching the upper extremity, for instance, the student may begin with the statement, "The upper extremity must be able to move in many different directions to be able to reach up (flexion), reach backward (extension), reach to the side (abduction), bring the arm back (adduction), or turn a screwdriver (pronation/supination)." Because of the need for the upper extremity to move in all these directions, the joint between the trunk and arm must be very versatile. Thus, the shoulder joint is a ball-and-socket joint to allow the movement in the different directions required. Further, the shallower the socket is, the more mobility the joint has. However, the versatility of the joint makes its dislocation easier.
2. **Given the anatomical description of a body part, what is its function?**
    This is the counterpart to the previous question regarding the relation between function and structure. The student should try to be imaginative

and not just accept the "textbook" information. One should be inquisitive, perceptive, and discriminating. For example, a student might speculate about why bone marrow is in the middle of bones instead of the bones being solid. The student might speculate as follows: "The main purpose of bones is to support the body and protect various organs. If the bones were solid, they might be slightly stronger, but they would be much heavier and be a detriment to the body. Also, production of blood cells is a critical function of the body. Thus, by having the marrow within the center of the bone, the process is protected."

3. **Given a patient's symptoms, what structure is affected?**

This is one of the most critical questions of clinical anatomy. It is also one of the major questions a clinician must answer when evaluating a patient. In clinical problem solving, the physician elicits information by asking questions (taking the history) and performing a physical examination while making observations. The history is the single most important tool for making a diagnosis. A thorough understanding of the anatomy aids the clinician tremendously because most diseases affect body parts under the skin and require "seeing under the skin." For example, the clinical data may be: "a 45-year-old woman complains of numbness of the perineal area and has difficulty voiding." The student may go through the following thinking process: "The sensory innervation of the perineal area is through sacral nerves S2 through S4, and control of the bladder is through the parasympathetic nerves, also S2 through S4. Therefore, two possibilities are a spinal cord problem involving those nerve roots or a peripheral nerve lesion. The internal pudendal nerve innervates the perineal region and is involved with micturition." Further information is supplied: "The patient states that she has had back pain since falling down 2 weeks ago." Now the lesion can be isolated to the spine, most likely the cauda equina (horse's tail), which is a bundle of spinal nerve roots traversing through the cerebrospinal fluid.

4. **Which lymph nodes are most likely to be affected by cancer at a particular location?**

The lymphatic drainage of a particular region of the body is important because cancer may spread through the lymphatics, and lymph node enlargement may occur due to infection. The clinician must be aware of these pathways to know where to look for metastasis (spread) of cancer. For example, if a cancer is located on the vulva labia majora (or the scrotum in the male), the most likely lymph node involved is the superficial inguinal nodes. The clinician would then be alert to palpating the inguinal region for lymph node enlargement, which would indicate an advanced stage of cancer and a worse prognosis.

5. **If an injury occurs to one part of the body, what is the expected clinical manifestation?**

If a laceration, tumor, trauma, or bullet causes injury to a specific area of the body, it is important to know which crucial bones, muscles, joints, vessels, and nerves might be involved. Also, based on experience, the clinician is aware of particular vulnerabilities. For example, the thinnest part of the skull is located in the temple region, and underneath this is the middle meningeal artery. Thus, a blow to the temple region may be disastrous. A laceration to the middle meningeal artery would lead to an epidural hematoma because this artery is located superficial to the dura and can cause cerebral damage.

6. **Given a deficit such as weakness or numbness, what other symptoms or signs would the patient most likely have?**

This requires a three-step process in analysis. First, the student must be able to deduce the initial injury based on the clinical findings. Second, a determination must be made of the probable site of injury. Third, the student must make an educated guess as to which other structures are in close proximity and, if injured, what the clinical manifestations would be. To be more skilled in learning these relations, one can begin from a clinical finding, propose an anatomical deficit, propose a mechanism or location of the injury, identify another nerve or vessel or muscle in that location, propose the new clinical finding, and so on.

7. **What is the male or female homologue to the organ in question?**

This knowledge of homologous correlates is important to understand the embryologic relations and, hence, the resultant anatomical relations. By being aware of the female and male homologues, fewer structures need to be memorized because analogous relations are easier to learn than two separate structures. For example, the vascular supplies of homologous structures are usually similar. The ovarian arteries arise from the abdominal aorta below the renal arteries; likewise, the testicular arteries arise from the abdominal aorta.

KEY POINTS

- The student should approach an anatomical structure by visualizing the structure and understanding its function.
- A standard anatomical position is used as a reference for anatomical planes and terminology of movement.
- There are seven key questions to stimulate the application of basic science information to the clinical arena.

REFERENCE

Moore KL, Dalley AF. Clinically oriented anatomy, 5th ed. Baltimore, MD: Lippincott Williams & Wilkins, 2006.

Clinical Cases

A 32-year-old woman delivered a large (4800 g) baby vaginally after some difficulty with her labor. Her prenatal course was complicated by diabetes, which occurred during pregnancy. At delivery, the infant's head emerged, but the shoulders were "stuck" behind the maternal symphysis pubis, requiring the obstetrician to apply some effort and maneuvers to free up the infant's shoulders and complete the delivery. The infant was noted to have a good cry and pink color but was not moving its right arm.

◆ **What is the most likely diagnosis?**

◆ **What is the most likely etiology for this condition?**

◆ **What is the likely anatomical mechanism for this disorder?**

ANSWERS TO CASE 1: BRACHIAL PLEXUS INJURY

Summary: A large (4800 g) infant of a diabetic mother is delivered after some difficulty and cannot move its right arm. There is a shoulder dystocia (the infant's shoulders are stuck after delivery of the head).

◆ **Most likely diagnosis:** Brachial plexus injury, probably Erb palsy

◆ **Most likely etiology for this condition:** Stretching of the upper brachial plexus during delivery

◆ **Likely anatomical mechanism for this disorder:** Stretching of nerve roots C5 and C6 by an abnormal increase in the angle between the neck and the shoulder

CLINICAL CORRELATION

During delivery, particularly of a large infant, shoulder dystocia may occur. In this situation, the fetal head emerges, but the shoulders become wedged behind the maternal symphysis pubis. An obstetrician will use maneuvers such as flexion of the maternal hips against the maternal abdomen (McRobert maneuver) or fetal maneuvers such as pushing the fetal shoulders into an oblique position. These actions are designed to allow delivery of the fetal shoulders without excessive traction on the fetal neck. Despite such carefully executed maneuvers, infants may be born with stretch injuries to the brachial plexus, resulting in nerve palsies. The most common of these is an upper brachial plexus stretch injury in which nerve roots C5 and C6 are affected, resulting in the infant's arm being limp and to its side. Most such injuries resolve spontaneously.

APPROACH TO THE BRACHIAL PLEXUS

Objectives

1. Be able to describe the spinal cord segments, named terminal branches, and the motor and sensory deficits of an **upper brachial plexus injury.**
2. Be able to describe the mechanism, spinal cord segments, named terminal branches, and the motor and sensory deficits of a **lower brachial plexus injury**.
3. Be able to describe the mechanism, spinal cord segments, named terminal branches, and the motor and sensory deficits with **cord injury** of the brachial plexus.

Definitions

Brachial plexus: A major peripheral nerve network formed by the anterior primary rami of the fifth cervical to the first thoracic spinal nerves.

Upper brachial plexus injury: Typically involves nerve roots C5 and C6, resulting in the upper limb hanging at the side, with medial rotation and the palm facing posteriorly.

Lower brachial plexus injury: Less common injury involving C8 through T1 and the ulnar nerve, leading to interosseous muscle atrophy and claw hand.

Shoulder dystocia: Condition whereby the fetal head delivers vaginally, but the shoulders are impacted behind the maternal bony pelvis.

DISCUSSION

The **brachial plexus** arises from the inferior portion of the cervical spinal cord enlargement. It is formed by the ventral **primary rami of spinal nerves C5 through C8** and most of **T1.** The network of nerves that form the brachial plexus is divided anatomically from proximal (medial) to distal (lateral) into **roots, trunks, divisions, cords,** and **terminal branches** (mnemonic: **Randy Travis Drinks Cold Texas Beer**). The roots of the plexus emerge from between the anterior and middle scalene muscles together with the subclavian artery. Arising from the roots are branches to the **longus colli and scalene muscles and the dorsal scapular and long thoracic nerves.** The roots unite to form **superior, middle,** and **inferior trunks.** The **suprascapular nerve** and the nerve to the **subclavius muscle** arise from the **superior trunk.** Each trunk is divided into **anterior** and **posterior divisions,** which will innervate musculature of the anterior and posterior compartments, respectively (Figure 1-1).

The anterior divisions of the superior and middle trunks unite to form the **lateral cord.** The **lateral cord** gives off the **lateral pectoral nerve.** The anterior division of the inferior trunk continues distally as the medial cord, whose branches are the **medial pectoral, medial brachial cutaneous,** and **medial antebrachial cutaneous nerves.** The posterior divisions of all three trunks unite to form the **posterior cord,** and its branches are the **upper** and **lower subscapular** and **thoracodorsal nerves.** The three cords are named for their relation to the **axillary artery,** which passes through the plexus at this level. The terminal branches of the brachial plexus are the **axillary, musculocutaneous, median, ulnar,** and **radial nerves.**

The **axillary nerve (C5** and **C6)** arises from the **posterior cord** and courses posteriorly around the **surgical neck of the humerus,** where it is at risk of injury. The **posterior circumflex humeral artery** accompanies the nerve in this course. The axillary nerve supplies the **deltoid** and **teres minor muscles,** is sensory to the skin over the lower portion of the deltoid, and is optimally tested on the **"shoulder patch"** portion of the upper arm. **Axillary nerve injury** such as by fracture at the **surgical neck of the humerus** results in an **inability to abduct the arm at the shoulder to a horizontal position** and **sensory loss in the shoulder patch area** (Figure 1-2).

The **musculocutaneous nerve (C5–C7)** is the continuation of the lateral cord. It courses distally through the coracobrachialis muscle to innervate it in

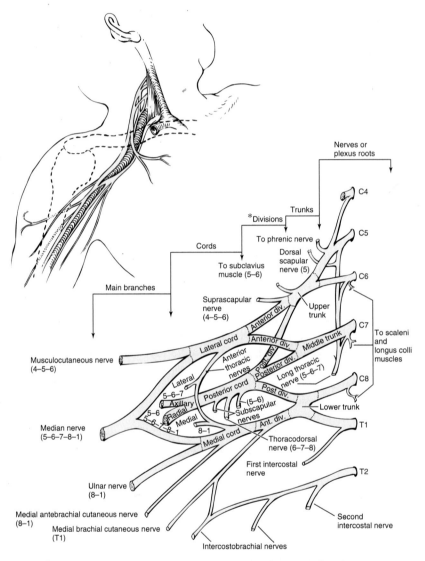

*Splitting of the plexus into anterior and posterior divisions is one of the most significant features in the redistribution of nerve fibers, because it is here that fibers supplying the flexor and extensor groups of muscles of the upper extremity are separated. Similar splitting is noted in the lumbar and sacral plexuses for the supply of muscles of the lower extremity.

Figure 1-1. The brachial plexus. (*Reproduced, with permission, from Waxman SG. Clinical Neuroanatomy, 25th ed. New York: McGraw-Hill, 2003:348.*)

Figure 1-2. The musculocutaneous nerves (C5 and C6) and axillary nerves (C5 and C6). (*Reproduced, with permission, from Waxman SG. Clinical neuroanatomy, 25th ed. New York: McGraw-Hill, 2003:350.*)

addition to the biceps brachii and brachialis muscles. The lateral antebrachial cutaneous nerve to the skin of the lateral forearm represents the terminal continuation of this nerve. Damage to the **musculocutaneous nerve** causes **weakness in supination and flexion of the shoulder and elbow.**

The upper portion of the brachial plexus arises from spinal cord segments C5 and C6, forms the **superior trunk,** and makes major contributions to the **axillary, musculocutaneous, lateral pectoral, and suprascapular nerves and the nerve to the subclavius muscle.** Injury to the upper plexus typically occurs with an increase in the angle between the shoulder and the neck. This can occur in a newborn during an obstetrical delivery or in adults as the result of a fall on the shoulder and side of the head and neck, which produces a widened angle. The resultant muscle paralysis due to such an injury may be understood more easily in an adult with such an injury. The **upper extremity hangs by the side** because the **deltoid and supraspinatus** (abductors of the arm) are paralyzed due to injury of the **axillary and suprascapular nerves,** respectively. In addition, the anterior deltoid, biceps brachii, and coracobrachialis (flexors of the arm) are paralyzed due to injury of the **axillary and musculocutaneous nerves.** The **elbow is extended and the hand is pronated due to paralysis of the biceps brachii and brachialis muscles,** both of which are innervated by the **musculocutaneous nerve.** The extremity is medially rotated due to paralysis of the teres minor and infraspinatus muscles (lateral rotators of the arm) and to injury to the axillary and suprascapular nerves. The palm of the hand is turned posteriorly in the **"waiter's tip" sign.** There is loss of sensation along the lateral aspect of the upper extremity, which corresponds to the **dermatome at C5 and C6.** The upper brachial plexus injury is known as **Erb or Erb-Duchenne palsy.**

The **ulnar nerve (C8 and T1)** is a continuation of the **medial cord,** which enters the posterior compartment through the medial intermuscular septum and passes distally to enter the forearm by curving posteriorly to the **medial epicondyle.** Here it is superficial and at risk of injury. It enters the anterior compartment of the forearm, where it innervates the **flexor carpi ulnaris and the bellies of the flexor digitorum profundus** to the **ring and little fingers.** The **ulnar nerve** enters the hand through a **canal (Guyon canal) superficial to the flexor retinaculum.** The nerve supplies all the **intrinsic muscles** of the **hand except** the **three thenar muscles and the lumbricals of the index and middle fingers.** It is sensory to the **medial border of the hand, the little finger, and the medial aspect of the ring finger.** Damage to the ulnar nerve in the upper forearm causes lateral (radial) deviation of the hand, with weakness in flexion and adduction of the hand at the wrist and loss of flexion at the distal interphalangeal joint of the ring and little fingers. Damage to the ulnar nerve in the upper forearm or at the wrist also results in loss of abduction and adduction of the index, middle, ring, and little fingers due to paralysis of the interossei muscles. **A "claw hand" deformity results,** and with longstanding damage, **atrophy of the interosseous muscles** occurs.

Injury to the **lower brachial plexus, known as Klumpke palsy,** occurs by a similar mechanism, that is, an abnormal widening of the angle between the upper extremity and the thorax. This may occur at obstetrical delivery by traction on the fetal head or when an individual reaches out to interrupt a fall. The roots from **C8 and T1** and/or the inferior trunk are stretched or torn. Spinal cord segments **C8 and T1 form the ulnar nerve** and a significant portion of the **median nerve.** The majority of the **muscles of the anterior forearm** is **innervated by the median nerve** (see Case 4) and will display weakness. Most of the **muscles of the hand** are innervated by the **ulnar nerve.** There will be loss of **sensation** along the **median aspect of the arm, forearm, hypothenar eminence,** and **little finger (C8 and T1 dermatome).**

Compression of the brachial plexus cords may occur with prolonged **hyperabduction** while performing overhead tasks. The **hyperabduction syndrome of pain** down the arm, **paresthesia, hand weakness,** and **skin redness,** may result from compression of the cords between the **coracoid process and pectoralis minor.** An **axillary-type crutch** that is too long can compress the posterior cord, leading to radial nerve palsy.

COMPREHENSION QUESTIONS

[1.1]   A 12-year-old boy is diagnosed with an upper brachial plexus injury after falling from a tree. He presents with his right upper arm at his side due to loss of abduction. Which of the following muscles are primarily responsible for abduction of the arm at the shoulder?

   A. Deltoid and biceps brachii
   B. Deltoid and supraspinatus
   C. Deltoid and infraspinatus
   D. Supraspinatus and infraspinatus
   E. Coracobrachialis and supraspinatus

[1.2]   Injury to the lateral cord of the brachial plexus will also injure its continuation, the musculocutaneous nerve. Which of the following findings would you observe in a patient with this injury?

   A. Weakness of abduction of the arm at the shoulder
   B. Weakness of adduction of the arm at the shoulder
   C. Weakness of extension of the forearm at the elbow
   D. Weakness of flexion of the forearm at the elbow
   E. Weakness of supination of the forearm and hand

[1.3]   A 22-year-old man is brought into the emergency department with a knife injury to the axilla. The physician suspects injury to the lower brachial plexus. Which of the following nerves is most likely to be affected?

   A. Axillary
   B. Musculocutaneous
   C. Vagus
   D. Radial
   E. Ulnar

Answers

[1.1] **B.** The deltoid and supraspinatus muscles, which are innervated by the axillary and suprascapular nerves, respectively, are the primary abductors of the arm at the shoulder.

[1.2] **D.** Injury to the musculocutaneous nerve will result in loss or weakness of flexion at the elbow due to paralysis of the biceps brachii and brachialis muscles.

[1.3] **E.** The C8 and T1 portions of the lower brachial plexus make up the majority of the ulnar nerve.

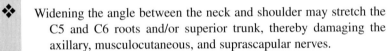

ANATOMY PEARLS

❖ Widening the angle between the neck and shoulder may stretch the C5 and C6 roots and/or superior trunk, thereby damaging the axillary, musculocutaneous, and suprascapular nerves.

❖ An upper plexus injury results in Erb palsy, which is characterized by an adducted and medially rotated arm, extended elbow, and pronated hand (waiter's tip sign).

❖ The axillary nerve is at risk from fractures of the surgical neck of the humerus.

❖ The musculocutaneous nerve supplies all the muscles of the anterior compartment of the arm.

❖ An abnormal increase in the angle between the upper limb and thorax and/or severe abduction traction may stretch the C8 and T1 roots and/or the inferior trunk and, hence, affect the ulnar and median nerves.

❖ A lower plexus injury may result in Klumpke palsy, which is characterized primarily by signs of ulnar nerve damage (claw hand).

❖ The ulnar nerve innervates all but five muscles of the hand: the three thenar muscles and the lumbricals to the index and middle fingers. In ulnar nerve palsies, the patent is unable to abduct and adduct the fingers.

❖ A posterior cord injury results in signs of radial nerve damage (wrist drop).

REFERENCES

Moore KL, Dalley AF. Clinically Oriented Anatomy, 5th ed. Baltimore, MD: Lippincott Williams & Wilkins, 2006:760–1, 773–81.
Netter FH. Atlas of Human Anatomy, 4th ed. Philadelphia, PA : Saunders, 2006: plates 430, 474. 477.
Snell RS. Clinical Anatomy by Regions, 8th ed. Baltimore, MD : Lippincott Williams & Wilkins, 2008:446–53, 536–7.

❖ CASE 2

A 32-year-old man is involved in a motor vehicle accident. He used three-point restraints and was driving a sedan. The driver of a pick-up truck ran a stop sign while going at approximately 45 mph and "T-boned" the patient's vehicle on the driver's side. The patient has multiple injuries including a displaced fracture of the left humerus. He complains of an inability to open his left hand and loss of sensation to a portion of his left hand.

◆ **What is the most likely diagnosis?**

◆ **What is the likely mechanism of the injury?**

◆ **What portion of the left hand is likely to have sensory deficit?**

ANSWERS TO CASE 2: RADIAL NERVE INJURY

Summary: A 32-year-old man is involved in a motor vehicle accident that causes a displaced fracture of the left humerus. He has motor and sensory losses to his left hand.

◆ **Most likely diagnosis:** Injury to the radial nerve as it spirals around the humerus, resulting in an inability to extend the wrist or fingers and loss of sensation of the hand

◆ **Likely mechanism:** Stretch or crush injury to the radial nerve as it spirals around the midshaft of the humerus

◆ **Likely location of sensory deficit:** Radial (lateral) side of the dorsum of the hand and dorsum of the thumb and index and middle digits

CLINICAL CORRELATION

The radial nerve is at particular risk of injury in its course in the radial groove as it spirals around the midshaft of the humerus. Humeral fractures involving the midshaft region are of particular concern. There is loss of innervation of the posterior extensor muscles in the forearm, resulting in wrist drop and an inability to extend the digits at the metacarpophalangeal joints. The sensory loss on the dorsum of the hand and digits reflects the distal cutaneous distribution of the radial nerve. The triceps muscle (extensor of the elbow) is typically spared; however, the patient usually will not attempt to move the limb due to pain from the fracture. The deep brachial artery has the same path as the radial nerve in the radial groove and has a similar risk for injury.

APPROACH TO THE RADIAL NERVE

Objectives

1. Be able to describe the origin, course, muscles innervated, and distal cutaneous regions supplied by the radial nerve.
2. Be able to describe the arterial blood supply to the upper limb.
3. Be able to describe the origin, course, muscles innervated, and distal cutaneous regions supplied by the five major terminal branches of the brachial plexus (Cases 1, 2, and 4).

Definitions

Fracture: A break in the normal integrity of a bone or cartilage.
Blunt trauma: Injury due to a crushing force as opposed to a sharp penetrating force.

DISCUSSION

The **radial nerve** is a continuation of the **posterior cord of the brachial plexus**, and it reaches the posterior compartment of the arm by coursing around the **radial groove** of the **humerus** with the **deep brachial artery** (Figure 2-1). It gives off multiple muscular branches to the **triceps muscle** in the posterior compartment. The nerve then pierces the lateral intermuscular septum to return to the anterior compartment of the arm and descends to the level of the lateral epicondyle of the humerus; at this level, it lies deep to the **brachio-radialis muscle,** where it divides into its two terminal branches. The **deep branch of the radial nerve is entirely motor to the muscles of the posterior compartment** of the **forearm.** The other terminal branch, the **superficial branch of the radial nerve,** is sensory to the dorsum of the hand and to the dorsum of the thumb, index finger, and the radial side of the middle finger. The radial nerve also has cutaneous **sensory branches to the posterior and lateral arm and to the posterior forearm.**

The **blood supply to the upper limb** is derived from the **brachial artery,** a direct continuation of the **axillary artery.** It begins at the lower border of the teres major muscle and accompanies the median nerve on the **medial aspect of the humerus,** where its pulsations can be palpated or the artery occluded to control hemorrhage. In its descent toward the elbow, it gives off the **deep brachial artery,** which supplies the posterior compartment of the arm, and **passes around the radial groove of the humerus** with the radial nerve. It also has **ulnar collateral branches to the elbow joint.** The **brachial artery** shifts anteriorly as it enters the forearm, lying **just medial to the tendon of the biceps brachii muscle in the cubital fossa.** At about the level of the neck of the radius, it divides into the ulnar and radial arteries, the main arteries of the forearm and hand. Near their origin, each sends recurrent arterial branches to supply the elbow joint.

The **radial artery** supplies the **lateral aspects of the forearm** and at the wrist passes dorsally (deep) through the **anatomical snuff box** (see Case 3) to become the **deep palmar arch.** The **ulnar artery** is the larger branch of the brachial, and it supplies the **medial aspect of the forearm.** A branch close to its origin, the common interosseous artery, divides into anterior and posterior interosseous arteries. The latter artery is the main blood supply to the posterior compartment. At the wrist, the **ulnar artery** enters the hand to form the **superficial palmar arch.** The **superficial and deep palmar arches** form an **arterial anastomosis** and give rise to **arteries to the digits.**

Also see Case 1.

Figure 2-1. The radial nerve. (*Reproduced, with permission, from Waxman SG. Clinical Neuroanatomy, 25th ed. New York: McGraw-Hill, 2003:351.*)

COMPREHENSION QUESTIONS

[2.1] An 18-year-old patient has been improperly fitted with axillary-type crutches, which have put pressure on the posterior cord of the brachial plexus. Which of the following terminal nerves would most likely be affected?

A. Axillary nerve
B. Musculocutaneous nerve
C. Median nerve
D. Radial nerve
E. Ulnar nerve

[2.2] A 24-year-old man is noted to have a midshaft humeral fracture after falling from a scaffold. Which of the following muscle tests would you perform to test the integrity of the radial nerve?

A. Flexion of the forearm at the elbow
B. Flexion of the hand at the wrist
C. Extension of the hand at the wrist
D. Abduction of the index, middle, ring, and little fingers
E. Adduction of the index, middle, ring, and little fingers

[2.3] A 45-year-old woman has a severe asthmatic exacerbation and requires an arterial blood gas specimen for management. If you are planning to draw the sample from the brachial artery, where should you insert the needle?

A. In the lateral aspect of the arm, between the biceps and triceps brachii muscles
B. Just lateral to the biceps tendon in the cubital fossa
C. Just medial to the biceps tendon in the cubital fossa
D. Just medial to the tendon of the flexor carpi radialis muscle at the wrist
E. Just lateral to the tendon of the flexor carpi ulnaris muscle at the wrist

Answers

[2.1] **D.** The radial nerve is a direct continuation of the posterior cord and is affected by injuries to the posterior cord.

[2.2] **C.** The radial nerve innervates the muscles of the posterior compartment, which contains the extensors of the wrist.

[2.3] **C.** The brachial artery lies superficial and just medial to the tendon of the biceps brachii in the cubital fossa.

ANATOMY PEARLS

 The radial nerve supplies all the muscles of the posterior compartment of the arm and forearm. Injury to the radial nerve results in wrist drop.

 The brachial artery lies immediately medial to the tendon of the biceps brachii muscle in the cubital fossa.

 The superficial and deep palmar arches are formed by the ulnar and radial arteries, respectively.

REFERENCES

Moore KL, Dalley AF. Clinically Oriented Anatomy, 5th ed. Baltimore, MD: Lippincott Williams & Wilkins, 2006:791–2, 832–4.

Netter FH. Atlas of Human Anatomy, 4th ed. Philadelphia, PA: Saunders, 2006: plates 432, 477–8.

Snell RS. Clinical Anatomy by Regions, 8th ed. Baltimore, MD: Lippincott Williams & Wilkins, 2008:450, 453, 457–9.

A 23-year-old male reports that he was playing "hoops" with friends from college, tripped as he was driving to the basket, and fell on his outstretched right hand with the palm down. Two days later, he phoned his anatomist father and related that his right wrist was painful. Later that day, he visited his father who noted that the wrist was slightly swollen, tender, but without deformity. He instructed his son to extend the right thumb, thereby accentuating the anatomical "snuff box," which is extremely tender to deep palpation. His father told him a radiograph is needed.

◆ **What is the most likely diagnosis?**

◆ **What is the most likely anatomic defect?**

ANSWERS TO CASE 3: WRIST FRACTURE

Summary: A 23-year-old male trips while playing basketball and suffers trauma to the right wrist. The wrist is slightly swollen, tender, but not deformed. However, deep palpation of the anatomical snuff box elicits extreme tenderness.

◆ **Most likely diagnosis:** Wrist fracture

◆ **Most likely anatomical defect:** Fracture of the narrow middle portion of the scaphoid carpal bone

CLINICAL CORRELATION

This young man tripped while playing basketball and stretched out his right hand to protect himself. His hand, with the palm down and probably deviated to the side of the radius, took the brunt of the fall, resulting in significant impact force to the wrist. This results in pain and swelling of the wrist, especially on the radial side, with **point tenderness deep in the anatomical snuff box.** This is the common mechanism for a **fracture of the scaphoid carpal bone**, the most commonly fractured carpal bone. Point tenderness over a bone or bony process is a hallmark of a fracture at that site. Radiologic confirmation of a fracture is important. The scaphoid bone has a unique blood supply, and proper reduction and alignment of the segments is necessary to decrease the risk of **avascular necrosis**. A fall on an outstretched hand in a way that produces hyperextension of the wrist may result in dislocation of the lunate bone. The lunate is usually displaced anteriorly into the carpal tunnel and may impinge on the median nerve. The lunate is the most commonly dislocated carpal bone. A fall on an outstretched palm may also result in a transverse fracture of the distal radius or a Colles fracture. A **Colles fracture** produces a dorsal displacement of the distal fragment, resulting in the characteristic **"dinner fork" deformity**. A Smith fracture of the radius in the same region of younger individuals is less common. In a **Smith fracture,** there is trauma to the dorsal aspect of a flexed wrist, and the wrist is deformed with the distal radial fragment displaced ventrally in a **"spade" deformity**.

APPROACH TO THE WRIST

Objectives

1. Be able to describe the bones and joints of the wrist.
2. Be able to describe the anatomy of the radius and ulnar as it relates to the transmission of forces in the upper limb and its effect on the forearm bones.
3. Be able to describe the boundaries of the anatomical snuff box and its clinical significance.

Definitions

Anatomical snuff box: Depression on the lateral aspect of the wrist formed by the tendons of the extensor pollicis brevis and abductor pollicis longus anteriorly and the extensor pollicis longus posteriorly.

Fracture: A break in the normal integrity of a bone or cartilage.

Avascular necrosis: Death of cells, tissues, or an organ due to insufficient blood supply.

DISCUSSION

The junction of the forearm and hand, called the **wrist region,** is a complex of several joints. The articulation of the distal radius with the ulna, called the **distal radioulnar joint,** is the site of movement of the radius anteriorly around the ulna during pronation. The **radius and ulna are united by an articular disc or triangular fibrocartilage** and associated ligaments, which intervenes between the ulna and carpal bones. The **wrist joint proper** is formed between the **distal radius,** the **triangular fibrocartilage,** and the **proximal row of carpal bones.** The **eight carpal bones** are arranged in proximal and distal rows of four bones each. From lateral to medial, the proximal row is composed of the **scaphoid, lunate, triquetrum, pisiform,** and the distal row of the **trapezium, trapezoid, capitate, hamate** (mnemonic: **some ladies try perfume that they can't handle).** Approximately 50 percent of movement at the wrist occurs at the wrist joint proper, with the remaining 50 percent occurring at the intercarpal joint, between the two rows of carpal bones. A capsule, reinforced by palmar and dorsal radiocarpal ligaments, surrounds the joint. The **radial collateral ligament** strengthens the capsule laterally and limits adduction (ulnar deviation). The **ulnar collateral ligament** strengthens the capsule medially and limits abduction (radial deviation) (Figure 3-1).

In addition to the distal radioulnar joint, the proximal radioulnar joint allows pivot movement of the radius with the humerus and the ulna during pronation and supination. The **radius and ulna are also joined by the interosseous membrane and its fibers to form a syndesmosis.** The individual fibers are attached proximally on the radius but distally on the ulna. **Impact forces on an outstretched hand are transmitted at the wrist to the radius, through the interosseous membrane to the ulna,** to the **humerus,** and then to the **shoulder,** which is attached to the trunk primarily by muscle. In this fashion, impact forces are transferred distally in the upper limb, with dissipation of the forces as they move proximally. A fall on an outstretched hand may cause fracture of the **radial head** under the right circumstances. Fracture of one forearm bone frequently results in dislocation of the other bone through forces transferred by the **interosseous membrane.**

wrist → radius → interosseous membrane → ulna → humerus

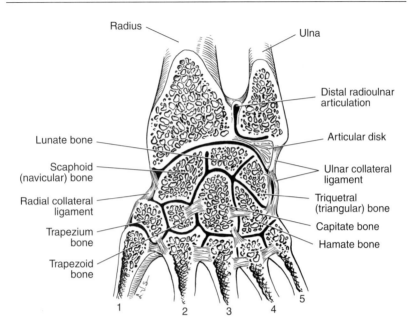

Figure 3-1. Articulations of the bones of the wrist. (*Reproduced, with permission, from Lindner HH. Clinical Anatomy. East Norwalk, CT:Appleton & Lange, 1989:563.*)

The **anatomical snuff box** is bounded anteriorly by the tendons of the **abductor pollicis longus** and the **extensor pollicis brevis** and posteriorly by the **tendon of the extensor pollicis longus**. The **scaphoid bone** and the **radial artery** (a branch of which supplies the scaphoid) lie in the floor of the snuff box.

COMPREHENSION QUESTIONS

[3.1]   A 23-year-old accountant trips over a briefcase and falls onto his outstretched hand. A carpal bone fracture is suspected. Which of the following bones is most likely fractured?

A. Scaphoid
B. Lunate
C. Triquetrum
D. Pisiform
E. Capitate

[3.2]   You are examining a radiograph of a patient's wrist and note malalign-
        ment (dislocation) of one of the carpal bones. Which of the following
        is most likely to be the dislocated carpal bone?

        A. Scaphoid
        B. Lunate
        C. Triquetrum
        D. Capitate
        E. Hamate

[3.3]   A patient with a severe tear of the medial collateral ligament of the
        wrist would likely display which of the following increased wrist
        movements?

        A. Flexion
        B. Extension
        C. Abduction
        D. Adduction
        E. Pronation

[3.4]   A 24-year-old male slips on a banana peel and falls onto his out-
        stretched hand. Which of the following structures transmits the force
        from the radius to the ulna?

        A. Triangular fibrocartilage
        B. Interosseous membrane
        C. Scaphoid bone
        D. Ulnar collateral ligament
        E. Radial collateral ligament

Answers

[3.1]   **A.** The scaphoid bone is the most frequently fractured carpal bone.

[3.2]   **B.** The lunate bone is the most frequently dislocated carpal bone.

[3.3]   **C.** The medial or ulnar collateral ligament limits abduction or radial
        deviation of the wrist, which would be increased if the ligament were
        severely torn.

[3.4]   **B.** The interosseous membrane conducts force from the radius to the
        ulna when the force originates from the wrist.

ANATOMY PEARLS

 The union at the distal radioulnar joint is formed by the triangular fibrocartilage.

 The chief bony articulation at the wrist is between the distal head of the radius and the proximal row of carpal bones.

❖ The interosseous membrane forms a fibrous joint between the radius and ulna, which is important for the transfer and dissipation of impact forces.

❖ The most commonly fractured and dislocated carpal bones are the scaphoid and lunate, respectively.

REFERENCES

Moore KL, Dalley AF. Clinically Oriented Anatomy, 5th ed. Baltimore, MD: Lippincott Williams & Wilkins, 2006:736–8.

Netter FH. Atlas of Human Anatomy, 4th ed. Philadelphia, PA: Saunders, 2006: plates 455–7.

Snell RS. Clinical Anatomy by Regions, 8th ed. Baltimore, MD: Lippincott Williams & Wilkins, 2008:480–1.

❖ CASE 4

A 34-year-old pregnant woman complains of tingling of her right index and middle fingers over a 2-month duration. She notes some weakness of her right hand and has begun to drop items such as her coffee cup. She has otherwise been healthy and denies any trauma or neck pain.

◆ **What is the most likely diagnosis?**

◆ **What is the anatomic mechanism for this condition?**

ANSWERS TO CASE 4: CARPAL TUNNEL SYNDROME

Summary: A pregnant woman has tingling and weakness of her right index and middle fingers.

◆ **Most likely diagnosis:** Carpal tunnel syndrome

◆ **Anatomical mechanism:** Compression of the medial nerve as it passes through the carpal tunnel of the wrist

CLINICAL CORRELATION

The most likely cause for this individual's symptoms is carpal tunnel syndrome. The carpal tunnel is a confined, rigid space at the wrist that contains nine tendons with their synovial sheaths and the median nerve. Any condition that further reduces the available space within the tunnel may compress the median nerve, producing numbness and pain in the areas of cutaneous distribution, muscle weakness (especially in the thumb), and muscle atrophy after long-term compression. However, we are not given the distribution of neuropathy of this case. The median nerve may be compressed in several sites along its length between the brachial plexus and the hand, but the carpal tunnel is the most common site. Carpal tunnel syndrome has been associated with endocrine conditions such as diabetes, hypothyroidism, hyperthyroidism, acromegaly, and pregnancy. Other causes include autoimmune disease, lipomas within the canal, hematomas, and carpal bone abnormalities. Females are more commonly affected than males in a ratio of 3:1. Initial treatment is a nighttime splint of the wrist and avoidance of excessive activity with the hand. If symptoms do not decrease, division of the flexor retinaculum (carpal tunnel release) may be necessary.

APPROACH TO THE CARPAL TUNNEL

Objectives

1. Be able to describe the structures that form and pass through the carpal tunnel.
2. Be able to describe the course, branches, and muscles innervated by the median nerve in the forearm and hand.
3. Be able to describe the skin areas supplied by the median nerve in the hand.
4. Be able to describe the course of the ulnar nerve at the wrist as it relates to the carpal tunnel.

Definitions

Neuropathy: Any disease or disorder of the peripheral nervous system.

Carpal tunnel syndrome: Entrapment of the median nerve within the carpal tunnel, resulting in pain, sensory paresthesia, and muscle weakness.

Muscle atrophy: Wasting of muscle tissue, often the result of disuse secondary to interference with its motor innervation.

DISCUSSION

The **carpal tunnel** is formed **posteriorly by the concave surfaces of the carpal bones** (see Case 3 for their anatomic arrangement). The **anterior boundary of the tunnel** is formed by a thickening of the deep fascia, the **flexor retinaculum** (transverse carpal ligament). The flexor retinaculum is attached laterally to the tubercles of the scaphoid and trapezium and medially to the **pisiform and hook of the hamate.** The carpal tunnel is a passageway for the **nine tendons and their investing synovial sheaths of the flexor muscles of the thumb and fingers:** four tendons each of the **flexor digitorum superficialis** (FDS) and **flexor digitorum profundus** (FDP), the **tendon of the flexor pollicis longus** (FPL), and the **median nerve.** The flexor retinaculum (and the extensor retinaculum dorsally) prevent "bowstringing" of the tendons of the extrinsic hand muscles at the wrist (Figure 4-1).

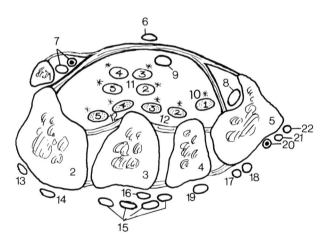

Figure 4-1. Carpal bones in cross section: 1 = pisiform, 2 = hamate, 3 = capitate, 4 = trapezoid, 5 = trapezium, 6 = palmaris longus, 7 = ulnar artery and vein, 8 = flexor carpi radialis, 9 = median nerve, 10 = flexor pollicis longus, 11 = flexor superficialis, 12 = flexor profundus, 13 = extensor carpi ulnaris, 14 = extensor digit minimi, 15 = extensor digitorum, 16 = extensor indicis, 17 = extensor carpi radialis brevis, 18 = extensor carpi radialis, 19 = extensor pollicis longus, 20 = radial artery, 21 = extensor pollicis brevis, 22 = abductor pollicis longus. (*Reproduced, with permission, from the University of Texas Health Science Center in Houston Medical School.*)

The **median nerve (C6 through T1)** is formed by contributions from the lateral and medial cords. It passes distally along the arm with the brachial artery and enters the cubital fossa **medial to that artery.** The nerve is at some risk in the **cubital fossa** region. It enters the forearm by passing between the heads of the **pronator teres muscle** and then descends in the forearm **between the FDS and the FDP.** In the forearm, the nerve innervates all the **muscles of the anterior compartment** except the flexor carpi ulnaris and the bellies of the FDP to the ring and little fingers. As it approaches the carpal tunnel at the wrist, the **median nerve lies just medial to the tendon of the flexor carpi radialis** muscle and slightly posterior to the tendon of the palmaris longus muscle, if it is present. The **median nerve** enters the hand through the carpal tunnel together with the tendons of the FDS, FDP, and FPL and is at risk of **laceration at the wrist** and of compression within the carpal tunnel, deep to the flexor retinaculum (transverse carpal ligament). Typically, the **recurrent branch of the median nerve** arises distal to the flexor retinaculum and the tunnel to innervate the **three thenar muscles: flexor pollicis brevis, abductor pollicis brevis, and the opponens pollicis.** The **lumbrical muscles of the index and middle fingers** receive their motor branches from adjacent common palmar digital branches.

The remainder of the median nerve divides into the **common palmar digital nerves** to the **skin of the thumb and the index, middle, and radial side of the ring fingers**, including their **dorsal nail beds**. The skin of the palm of the hand and thenar eminence is supplied by the palmar cutaneous branch of the median nerve, which typically arises from the median nerve in the distal forearm and does not traverse the carpal tunnel. **Intact skin sensation in the palm** of the hand suggests **carpal tunnel** entrapment of the median nerve, whereas **loss of palmar skin sensation** suggests a **higher nerve lesion**.

Damage to the median nerve in the upper forearm results in **loss of pronation, weakness in flexion at the wrist, and medial (ulnar) deviation.** There will also be **loss of flexion at the proximal interphalangeal joint of the index, middle, ring, and little fingers and loss of flexion at the distal interphalangeal joints of the index and middle fingers.** Damage to the **median nerve** in the **upper forearm** or at the wrist will also result in **loss of flexion, abduction and opposition of the thumb, and flexion at the metacarpal phalangeal joints of the index and middle fingers.** Loss of the median nerve results in the **"hand of benediction"** when the patient is asked to make a fist and an "ape hand" due to longstanding injury with atrophy of the thenar muscles (Figure 4-2).

The **ulnar nerve**, which innervates all the other intrinsic hand muscles not noted above, enters the hand **anterior to the flexor retinaculum** with and **medial to the ulnar artery**. The artery and nerve are covered anteriorly by a condensation of the fascia of the forearm, called the **volar carpal ligament**. Thus the ulnar nerve and artery come to lie in the **Guyon canal**, bounded anteriorly by the volar carpal ligament, posteriorly by the flexor retinaculum, medially by the pisiform, and laterally by the hook of the hamate.

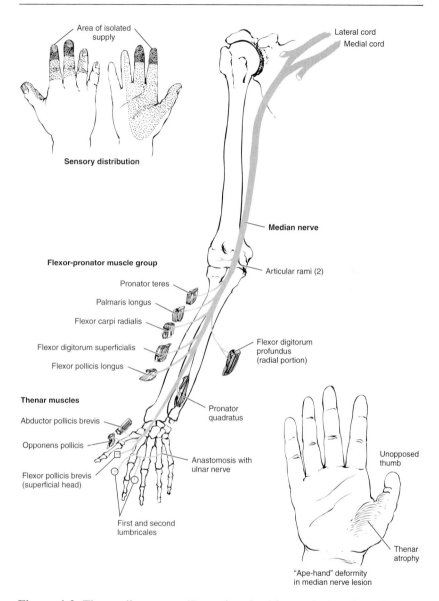

Figure 4-2. The median nerve. (*Reproduced, with permission, from Waxman SG. Clinical Neuroanatomy, 25th ed. New York: McGraw-Hill, 2003:352.*)

COMPREHENSION QUESTIONS

[4.1]   You are examining an axial (cross-section) magnetic resonance imaging (MRI) scan of the wrist and have identified the carpal tunnel. Which of the following is the structure that forms the anterior wall of the tunnel?

A. Palmar aponeurosis
B. Volar carpal ligament
C. Flexor retinaculum
D. Extensor retinaculum
E. Deep fascia

[4.2]   As you are explaining carpal tunnel syndrome to a woman who has the condition, shown where the median nerve is located just as it is about to enter the tunnel. Where is the median nerve located?

A. Just lateral to the flexor carpi radialis tendon
B. Must medial to the flexor carpi radialis tendon
C. Just medial to the flexor palmaris longus tendon
D. Just lateral to the flexor carpi ulnaris tendon
E. Just medial to the flexor carpi ulnaris tendon

[4.3]   If the median nerve were severed in an industrial accident at the wrist, which of the following muscles would still retain their function?

A. Flexor pollicis brevis
B. Abductor pollicis brevis
C. Opponens pollicis
D. Lumbricals of the index and middle fingers
E. Lumbricals of the ring and little fingers

Answers

[4.1]   **C.** The flexor retinaculum or transverse carpal ligament forms the anterior boundary of the carpal tunnel.

[4.2]   **B.** The median nerve lies just medial to the tendon of the flexor carpi radialis at the wrist.

[4.3]   **E.** The lumbricals to the ring and little finger are innervated by the ulnar nerve.

ANATOMY PEARLS

 All of the muscles of the anterior compartment of the forearm are supplied by the median nerve except the flexor carpi ulnaris and the medial half of the flexor digitorum profundus, which are innervated by the ulnar nerve.

 Injury to the median nerve results in the hand of benediction when attempting to make a fist.

 The carpal tunnel is formed by the flexor retinaculum and the eight carpal bones.

 The carpal tunnel contains nine tendons (four for the FDS, four for the FDP, and one for the FPL) and the median nerve.

The median nerve supplies five muscles in the hand (flexor pollicis brevis; abductor pollicis brevis; opponens pollicis; lumbricals 1 and 2); the skin of the thumb; index, middle, and lateral ring fingers.

 The palmar cutaneous branch of the median nerve does not traverse the carpal tunnel.

 The ulnar nerve does not traverse the carpal tunnel; it enters the hand anterior to the flexor retinaculum in Guyon canal.

REFERENCES

Moore KL, Dalley AF. Clinically Oriented Anatomy, 5th ed. Baltimore, MD: Lippincott Williams & Wilkins, 2006:819–22, 839–44.

Netter FH. Atlas of Human Anatomy, 4th ed. Philadelphia, PA: Saunders, 2006, plates 460–1, 475.

Snell RS. Clinical Anatomy by Regions, 8th ed. Baltimore, MD: Lippincott Williams & Wilkins, 2008:451, 500, 540.

A 17-year-old defensive end was attempting to tackle a fullback with an out-stretched left arm. The arm was hit with substantial force, and he now complains of severe shoulder pain and his left arm is hanging down with some external rotation. He does not move the limb due to the pain. A radiograph is negative for a fracture, but the head of the humerus is superimposed on the neck of the scapula.

◆ **What is the most likely diagnosis?**

◆ **What is the most likely nerve injured?**

ANSWERS TO CASE 5: SHOULDER DISLOCATION

Summary: A 17-year-old football player's left arm was outstretched and hit with some force. He has shoulder pain, and his arm hangs down his side with external rotation. There is no fracture, and the humeral head is superimposed on the scapular neck.

◆ **Most likely diagnosis:** Glenohumeral joint dislocation (shoulder dislocation)

◆ **Most likely nerve injured:** Axillary nerve

CLINICAL CORRELATION

The shoulder is the most commonly dislocated large joint of the body, and is most commonly dislocated in an anterior direction. Typically, the dislocation is also inferior such that the humeral head is located inferior and lateral to the coracoid process. The humeral head will often have an infraglenoid and infra-clavicular position. The diagnosis may be difficult to make. The typical mechanism is that of a violent force to the humerus that is abducted and externally rotated, resulting in extension of the joint; this action displaces the humeral head inferiorly, thus tearing the weak inferior portion of the shoulder joint capsule. This is facilitated by the fulcrum effect of the acromion. The strong flexor and adductor muscles pull the humeral head anteriorly and medially to the usual subcoracoid position. In general, the patient will not move the arm and will support the limb flexed at the elbow with the opposite hand. The arm will be slightly abducted and medially rotated. The usually rounded curve of the shoulder is lost, and there is a depression evident inferior to the acromion. The humeral head is palpable, if not visible, in the deltopectoral triangle. First priorities are assessment of the neural and vascular integrity of the upper limb by testing motor and sensory functions of the fingers and palpation of the radial pulse. Different methods to reduce the dislocation exist, including the modified Hippocratic method in which one operator pulls on a sheet placed around the thorax of the patient, while a second operator gently puts traction on the wrist of the affected side. Other injuries that may accompany a shoulder dislocation include strain on the tendons of the subscapularis and supraspinatus muscles, tears of the glenoid labrum, fracture of the greater tubercle of the humerus, trauma to the axillary nerve (as demonstrated by loss of sensation in the shoulder patch region over the deltoid muscle), and trauma to the axillary artery or its branches such as the posterior circumflex humeral or subscapular arteries.

APPROACH TO THE SHOULDER

Objectives

1. Be able to describe the bones and joints that make up the shoulder girdle.
2. Be able to delineate the anatomy of the glenohumeral joint.
3. Be able to list the extrinsic muscles of the shoulder, their action at the shoulder, and their innervation.
4. Be able to describe the components of the rotator cuff, their action, innervation, and their functional importance to the shoulder.

Definitions

Shoulder: Junction between the arm and the trunk.
Shoulder girdle: The clavicle, scapula, and proximal humerus.

DISCUSSION

The **shoulder girdle and shoulder joint** proper are composed of the **clavicle, scapula, and the proximal portion of the humerus.** The only bony articulation between the shoulder girdle and the trunk occurs at the sternoclavicular joint. This strong joint has two joint spaces created by a cartilage articular disc. The synovial articulation of the clavicle with the manubrium of the sternum is strengthened by a joint capsule, anterior and posterior sternoclavicular, and interclavicular and costoclavicular ligaments. The lateral end of the **clavicle** articulates with the **acromion of the scapula** to form the **acromioclavicular joint.** An incomplete articular disc is present within this synovial joint. A thin, loose capsule surrounds the acromioclavicular joint, which is reinforced superiorly by an **acromioclavicular ligament,** but its chief strength and support is derived from the **trapezoid and conoid ligaments,** which together form the **coracoclavicular ligament.**

The articulation of the **glenoid cavity** on the neck of the scapula with the head of the humerus forms the **glenohumeral joint.** This **shallow ball-and-socket synovial joint** forms the shoulder joint proper. The anatomy of this joint allows a **wide range of motion,** although **stability is decreased.** The diameter of the humeral head is about three times greater than the diameter of the glenoid cavity, which is increased somewhat by a rim of fibrocartilage attached to the margin of the glenoid, the **glenoid labrum.** The joint capsule attaches to the margin of the glenoid proximally and to the anatomical neck of the humerus distally. The **capsule has openings** for the tendon of the **long head of the biceps muscle** and **for the subscapular bursa,** which communicates with the joint cavity. **Three glenohumeral ligaments,** band-like thickenings of the anterior capsule, are identifiable only internally (Figure 5-1). The **coracohumeral ligament** reinforces the capsule superiorly, and the **transverse humeral ligament** bridges the **intertubercular groove** with the tendon and synovial sheath of the long head of the biceps brachii muscle. The **roof of**

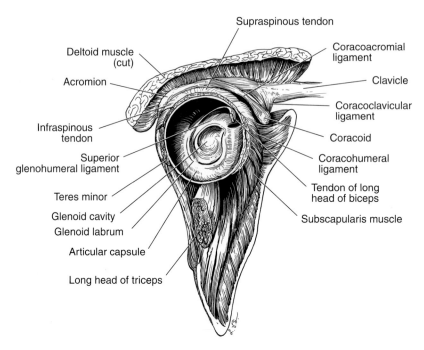

Figure 5-1. Anatomy of the shoulder joint. (*Reproduced, with permission, from Lindner HH. Clinical Anatomy. East Norwalk, CT: Appleton & Lange, 1989:528.*)

the glenohumeral joint is formed by the inferior surface of the **acromion** and **the coracoacromial ligament.**

The upper limb is attached to the trunk primarily by muscles. This group of muscles, the extrinsic muscles of the shoulder, originates from the trunk and inserts onto the scapula in most instances or the humerus directly. The action of muscles attaching to the scapula produces movement of the scapula, which greatly increases the range of motion at the shoulder. The extrinsic muscles and the action and innervation of each are listed in Table 5-1.

The **intrinsic muscles of the shoulder** originate from the scapula and insert onto the humerus. They include the **deltoid, teres major, and the rotator cuff muscles.** The **rotator cuff tendons** surround and blend with the capsule of the glenohumeral joint and provide **major strength and stability to the joint.** The intrinsic muscles of the shoulder and their actions and innervations are presented in Table 5-2. The tendon of the **supraspinatus muscle** passes **superior** to the capsule, between it and the acromion and deltoid muscle to insert onto the **greater tubercle.** The **subacromial (subdeltoid) bursa** intervenes between the tendon and the undersurface of the acromion and the deltoid muscle. Nevertheless, the **supraspinatus tendon** is typically damaged with rotator cuff tears.

Table 5-1

EXTRINSIC MUSCLES OF THE SHOULDER

MUSCLE	ACTION	INNERVATION
Trapezius	Retract, elevate, depress, rotate scapula	Spinal accessory nerve
Latissimus dorsi	Extend, adduct, medially rotate arm	Thoracodorsal nerve
Levator scapulae	Elevate, rotate scapula	Dorsal scapular nerve
Rhomboid major and minor	Retract and rotate scapula	Dorsal scapular nerve
Serratus anterior	Protract and rotate scapula	Long thoracic nerve
Pectoralis major	Adduct and medially rotate arm	Lateral and medial pectoral nerves
Pectoralis minor	Stabilizes scapula	Medial pectoral nerve

Table 5-2

INTRINSIC MUSCLES OF THE SHOULDER

MUSCLE	ACTION	INNERVATION
Deltoid	Abduct, flex, and extend arm	Axillary nerve
Teres major	Adducts and medially rotates arm	Lower subscapular nerve
Supraspinatus*	Initiates abduction of arm	Suprascapular nerve
Infraspinatus*	Laterally rotates arm	Suprascapular nerve
Teres minor*	Laterally rotates arm	Axillary nerve
Subscapularis*	Adducts and medially rotates arm	Upper and lower subscapular nerve

*Rotator cuff muscles

COMPREHENSION QUESTIONS

[5.1]   You are evaluating a radiograph of the only bony articulation between
        the upper limb and the trunk. Which of the following joints are you
        evaluating?

        A. Glenohumeral
        B. Acromioclavicular
        C. Humeroclavicular
        D. Coracoclavicular
        E. Sternoclavicular

[5.2]   You are explaining the anatomy of the shoulder to a young athlete who
        has sustained an injury to one of his shoulders. You tell him the chief
        stability to this joint is from which of the following?

        A. Glenohumeral ligaments
        B. Acromioclavicular ligament
        C. Rotator cuff muscles
        D. Coracoclavicular ligaments
        E. Coracohumeral ligament

[5.3]   A college baseball pitcher has shoulder discomfort and you suspect a
        rotator cuff tear. You will most likely see damage to the tendon of
        which of the following muscles?

        A. Supraspinatus
        B. Infraspinatus
        C. Subscapularis
        D. Teres major
        E. Teres minor

Answers

[5.1]   **E.** The upper limb is attached to the trunk only at the sternoclavicular
        joint. The primary attachment is muscular.

[5.2]   **C.** The primary stability to the glenohumeral joint is provided by the
        tendons of the rotator cuff.

[5.3]   **A.** The tendon of the supraspinatus is typically damaged in a rotator
        cuff tear due to the narrow space between the head of the humerus
        and the acromion.

ANATOMY PEARLS

❖ Shoulder dislocations are common, almost always anterior, and place the axillary nerve at risk.

❖ The only bony articulation between the upper limb and the trunk is at the sternoclavicular joint. The primary attachment of the limb to the trunk is by musculature.

❖ The shallow ball-and-socket glenohumeral joint permits a wide range of motion, but with decreased stability.

❖ The tendons of the rotator cuff muscles provide primary strength and stability to the glenohumeral joint.

❖ The supraspinatus muscle tendon blends with the superior capsule. Even though protected from the undersurface of the acromion by the subacromial (subdeltoid) bursa, its tendon is usually injured in rotator cuff tears.

REFERENCES

Moore KL, Dalley AF. Clinically Oriented Anatomy, 5th ed. Baltimore, MD: Lippincott Williams & Wilkins, 2006:760–3, 853–9.

Netter FH. Atlas of Human Anatomy, 4th ed. Philadelphia, PA: Saunders, 2006: plates 419–23.

Snell RS. Clinical Anatomy by Regions, 8th ed. Baltimore, MD: Lippincott Williams & Wilkins, 2008:462–5.

A 37-year-old male accountant is picked up by his wife at his office. He gets into the passenger seat of their automobile and turns to get the safety belt as his wife begins to exit the parking lot. Another vehicle entering the lot strikes their vehicle head on, and he is thrown forward by the sudden deceleration. His left knee strikes the dashboard violently, and he feels a painful pop in his left hip. After ambulance transport to the hospital emergency department, he is noted to have great pain in the left hip region. Compared with his right leg, he is noted to have a shortened left lower limb that is adducted and medially rotated. There is a painful mass in the lateral gluteal region.

◆ **What is the most likely diagnosis?**

◆ **What are the structures involved in this injury?**

◆ **What clinically important structures are at potential risk?**

ANSWERS TO CASE 6: POSTERIOR HIP DISLOCATION

Summary: A 37-year-old male automobile passenger was turning to his right during a head-on collision, in which his left knee struck the dashboard. He experiences a painful pop in his left hip. His left hip is very painful, and his left lower limb is shortened, adducted, and medially rotated. A large painful mass is present in the lateral gluteal area.

◆ **Most likely diagnosis:** Posterior hip dislocation, with or without acetabular fracture

◆ **Structures involved:** Hip joint, including the femoral head, joint capsule and ligaments, and acetabulum

◆ **Structures at risk:** Sciatic nerve

CLINICAL CORRELATION

This male automobile passenger has suffered a deceleration injury in which his left knee has forcefully impacted the vehicle's dashboard, forcing the femoral head posteriorly over the rim of the acetabulum. As he turned to reach for the safety belt, his hip was flexed by his sitting position, adducted and medially rotated, the classic hip position for this type of injury. The painful pop was the femoral head tearing through the posterior joint capsule and ligaments. The painful lateral gluteal mass is the femoral head on the lateral aspect of the ilium, and the limb appears short due to the abnormal position of the femoral head. The first step would be radiographic confirmation of the dislocation or dislocation fracture. This would be followed by urgent reduction of the dislocation to decrease the risk of avascular necrosis of the femoral head and other complications such as posttraumatic arthritis. Fracture repair, if present, may be performed at a later time.

APPROACH TO THE HIP JOINT

Objectives

1. Be able to describe the anatomy of the hip joint, including the proximal femur, joint capsule and ligaments, and acetabulum.
2. Be able to draw the sciatic nerve as it relates to the hip joint.

Definitions

Hip bone: Os coxae, irregular flat bone formed by the fusion of the pubis, ilium, and ischium.

Hip joint: Joint formed by the acetabulum and the head of the femur.

Sciatic nerve: The largest nerve of the body, formed from the sacral plexus by the ventral rami of L4 through S3, and anatomically unites the common fibular and tibial nerves.

DISCUSSION

The **hip joint** is a unique ball-and-socket joint formed by the femur and hip bone that combines stability for the transference of weight to the lower limbs and enables an erect posture, with a wide range of motion. The **ball portion** of the joint is formed by the **head of the femur** and is angled **superomedially** to the shaft by the neck. The large adjacent **greater and lesser trochanters** serve as points of attachment for muscles acting across the hip joint. The **socket** portion of the joint is formed by the **cup-shaped acetabulum** on the lateral surface of the hip bone (os coxae). The hip bone is formed by the fused **ilium, ischium, and pubic bones,** all of which participate in forming the **acetabulum.** The depth of the acetabulum is increased by a **C-shaped rim** of **fibrocartilage** called the **acetabular labrum.** The incomplete inferior portion of the labrum, the acetabular notch, is completed by the **transverse acetabular ligament,** and the weak, intra-articular **ligament of the femoral head** passes from the head to the acetabulum adjacent to the notch. The femoral head and acetabulum are covered with articular cartilage.

The **hip joint** is surrounded by a **capsule,** lined with a synovial membrane, and strengthened by three ligamentous thickenings, named for their proximal attachments. The capsule is reinforced anteriorly and superiorly by the strong, **inverted Y-shaped iliofemoral ligament.** Inferior and posterior capsular thickenings are the **pubofemoral and ischiofemoral ligaments,** respectively. The blood supply to the hip joint comes from the **lateral and medial circumflex arteries,** typically branches of the **deep femoral artery,** with the **medial circumflex artery being the most important.** These **vessels** reach the femoral head along the neck, where they are **at risk with femoral neck fractures.** A small artery of the head (a branch of the obturator artery) runs within the ligament of the head.

In addition to producing movement at the hip joint, the **muscles** crossing the joint impart much of the **joints' stability** while standing erect. The movements at the hip joint and the muscles (with their innervation) producing these movements are listed in Table 6-1.

The **large sciatic nerve** (Figure 6-1) exits the pelvis through the **greater sciatic foramen** and enters the **deep gluteal region** immediately **inferior to the piriformis muscle.** The sciatic nerve is actually the **combined common fibular nerve (lateral portion) and the tibial nerve (medial portion).** The common fibular nerve innervates the lateral compartment muscles (superficial fibular branch) and the anterior compartment muscles (deep fibular branch) of the leg. The **tibial portion innervates the muscles of posterior compartments of the thigh and leg (calf) and the sole of the foot.** The sciatic nerve lies **posterior to the hip joint**.

Table 6-1
MUSCLES ACTING ON THE HIP JOINT

	MUSCLES	INNERVATION
Flexion	Iliopsoas (psoas)	Anterior rami L1–3 nerves
	Iliopsoas (iliacus), rectus femoris, pectineus, sartorius	Femoral nerve
	Adductor longus, brevis, and magnus, gracilis	Obturator nerve
	Tensor fascia lata	Superior gluteal nerve
Extension	Hamstrings: semitendinosus, semimembranosus, long head biceps femoris, adductor magnus (hamstring portion)	Tibial portion of sciatic nerve
	Gluteus maximus	Inferior gluteal nerve
Abduction	Gluteus medius and minimus, tensor fascia lata	Superior gluteal nerve
Adduction	Adductor longus, brevis and magnus, gracilis, obturator externus	Obturator nerve
	Pectineus	Femoral nerve
Medial rotation	Gluteus medius and minimus, tensor fascia lata	Inferior gluteal nerve
Lateral rotation	Obturator internus, piriformis, superior and inferior gemelli, quadratus femoris	Direct nerves to muscles arising from L5, S1–2
	Obturator externus	Obturator nerve
	Gluteus maximus	Inferior gluteal nerve

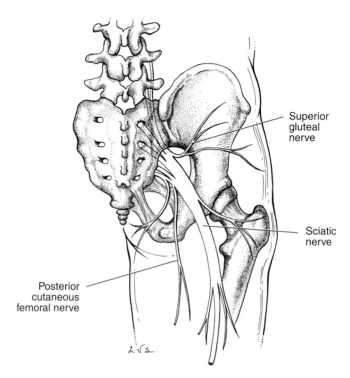

Figure 6-1. The sciatic nerve. (*Reproduced, with permission, from Lindner HH. Clinical Anatomy. East Norwalk, CT: Appleton & Lange, 1989:591.*)

COMPREHENSION QUESTIONS

[6.1]   In a patient who has a posterior dislocation of the hip, which of the following ligamentous structures would be torn?

A. Pubofemoral ligament
B. Iliofemoral ligament
C. Ischiofemoral ligament
D. Lacunar ligament
E. Sacrotuberous ligament

[6.2]   A 54-year-old man has just dislocated his right hip. The physician is concerned about the integrity of the joint's blood supply. Which artery is the main blood supply to the hip joint?

A. Lateral circumflex femoral
B. Medial circumflex femoral
C. Superficial circumflex iliac
D. Deep circumflex iliac
E. Perforating

[6.3]   A patient with the hip dislocation is also exhibiting weakness of exten-
         sion of the thigh at the hip. This would indicate possible damage to
         which of the following?

         A. Femoral nerve
         B. Obturator nerve
         C. Common fibular portion of the sciatic nerve
         D. Tibial portion of the sciatic nerve
         E. Saphenous nerve

Answers

[6.1]   **C.** Posterior dislocation of the hip would tear the ischiofemoral ligament,
         which reinforces the capsule of the hip posteriorly.

[6.2]   **B.** The chief blood supply to the hip is the medial circumflex femoral
         artery.

[6.3]   **D.** Most of the extensor muscles of the hip (the hamstrings) are inner-
         vated by the tibial portion of the sciatic nerve. The gluteus maximus
         muscle, innervated by the inferior gluteal nerve, could still weakly
         extend the thigh at the hip.

ANATOMY PEARLS

 The bones forming the hip bone, ilium, ischium, and pubis converge
    to form the acetabulum.
 The strongest ligament reinforcing the hip capsule is the iliofemoral
    or Y ligament.
 The most important artery supplying the hip joint is the medial cir-
    cumflex femoral artery.

REFERENCES

Moore KL, Dalley AF. Clinically Oriented Anatomy, 5th ed. Baltimore, MD:
    Lippincott Williams & Wilkins, 2006:619–23, 675–83.
Netter FH. Atlas of Human Anatomy, 4th ed. Philadelphia, PA: Saunders, 2006:
    plates 486–7. 503.
Snell RS. Clinical Anatomy by Regions, 8th ed. Baltimore, MD: Lippincott
    Williams & Wilkins, 2008, 587–92.

A 25-year-old woman is on her first ski trip to Colorado. She has advanced from the "bunny slopes" and, during the last run of the day, falls and twists her right leg. She cannot stand on her right leg due to pain and is brought down the hill in a snow mobile. On examination, the right knee is swollen and tender. With the patient sitting on the stretcher with her knee flexed, the lower leg seems to have several centimeters of excess anterior mobility.

◆ **What is the most likely diagnosis?**

◆ **What is the mechanism of the injury?**

ANSWERS TO CASE 7: ANTERIOR CRUCIATE LIGAMENT RUPTURE

Summary: A 25-year-old woman twists her right lower limb in a ski accident. She has right knee swelling, tenderness, and excessive anterior mobility with the knee flexed.

◆ **Most likely diagnosis:** Anterior cruciate ligament (ACL) tear

◆ **Mechanism of injury:** Excessive rotational force strains or ruptures the ligament

CLINICAL CORRELATION

Injuries to the knee are very common because it bears weight, combines mobility in flexion and extension, and allows some rotation. The stability of the knee depends entirely on its ligaments and muscles. Sports injuries to the knee are most commonly caused by high-speed and rotational forces applied to the leg through the knee joint. In addition, certain ligaments are anatomically related to the menisci, on which the distal femur articulates. This 25-year-old woman was involved in a ski injury, a common setting for ACL injury. The twisting force to the lower limb when a ski becomes lodged in snow and the body continues to rotate can produce significant trauma to the knee. The ACL passes from the posterior aspect of the distal femur to the intercondylar region of the anterior aspect of the proximal tibia; it limits anterior movement of the tibia in relation to the femur. Thus, on examination, this patient exhibits the "anterior drawer sign," or excessive anterior mobility of the tibia with the knee flexed. This injury will usually require surgical repair.

APPROACH TO THE KNEE JOINT

Objectives

1. Be able to describe the anatomy of the knee joint, including the bones, ligaments, possible movements, and the muscles responsible for these movements.
2. Be able to describe the mechanism of injury to the four main ligaments of the knee.

Definitions

Knee: Hinge joint between the femur and proximal tibia.
Patella: A triangular bone approximately 5 cm in diameter situated in the front of the knee at the insertion of the quadriceps tendons.
Meniscus: Crescent-shaped intra-articular cartilage.

DISCUSSION

The **knee joint** is a **synovial hinge joint** formed by the distal **femur, proximal tibia, and the patella.** It is a relatively stable joint; its movements consist primarily of flexion and extension, with some gliding, rolling, and locking rotation. The **distal femur** forms two large knuckle-like **lateral and medial condyles,** which articulate with **lateral and medial tibial condyles.** The superior surfaces of the tibial condyles are flattened to form the **tibial plateau.** An **intercondylar eminence** fits between the femoral condyles, and the proximal fibula articulates with the lateral tibial condyle but is not a part of the knee joint. The **patella** articulates with the femur anteriorly. The flat tibial condylar surfaces are modified to accommodate the femoral condyles by the **C-shaped lateral and medial menisci.** These fibrocartilaginous structures are wedge-shaped in cross section, being thick externally but thin internally, are firmly attached to the tibial condyles, and serve as shock absorbers. The **lateral meniscus** is the smaller of the two, being somewhat **circular,** whereas the **medial meniscus is C-shaped.** The femoral and remaining portions of the tibial condyles are covered with articular cartilage (Figure 7-1).

The knee joint is surrounded by a capsule, lined with synovial membrane, and reinforced by several ligamentous thickenings. Anteriorly, the **tendon of the quadriceps femoris muscle group has the patella embedded within it.** Inferior to the patella, the tendon becomes the patellar ligament, which inserts into the **tibial tuberosity.** Laterally, the capsule is thickened to form the **fibular (lateral) collateral ligament** from the lateral femoral epicondyle to the fibular head. The fibular collateral ligament remains separated from the lateral meniscus by the tendon of the popliteus muscle. It prevents increasing the lateral angle or adduction of the leg at the knee. The **tibial (medial or MCL) collateral ligament** extends from the medial femoral epicondyle to the medial tibial condyle. The deep aspect of this ligament is firmly attached to the margin of the medial meniscus. It prevents increasing the medial angle or abduction of the leg at the knee. Posteriorly, the capsule is reinforced by **oblique and arcuate popliteal ligaments.** The knee is unique due to the presence of two intra-articular ligaments, **the ACL and posterior cruciate ligament (PCL).** The cruciate ligaments are covered by synovial membrane and thus are external to the synovial cavity and are named by their attachment to the tibial. The ACL extends from the anterior tibial plateau near the intercondylar eminence to the posteromedial aspect of the lateral femoral condyle. It **limits anterior displacement of the tibial in relation to the femur** and limits hyperextension. The **PCL** extends from the posterior aspect of the tibial plateau to the anterolateral aspect of the medial femoral condyle. In its course, it crosses the ACL on its medial side and is **larger and stronger** than the ACL. The **PCL limits posterior displacement** of the tibia on the femur and limits hyperflexion. A dozen or so **bursae** are associated with the knee joint, and four of these communicate with the synovial cavity of the joint: suprapatellar, popliteus, anserine, and gastrocnemius. Thus, inflammation of any of these

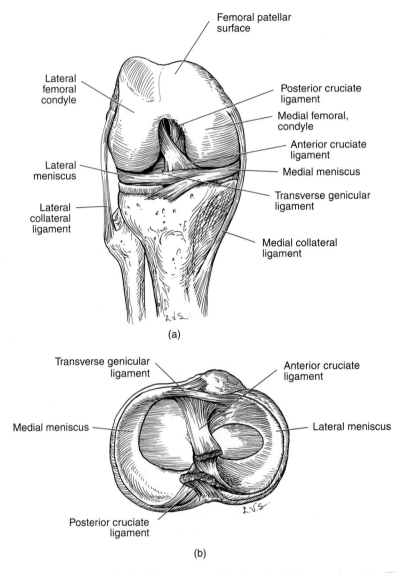

Figure 7-1. The knee joint. Ligaments of the knee in full extension (A). The superior aspect of the knee showing the menisci (B). (*Reproduced, with permission, from Lindner HH. Clinical Anatomy. East Norwalk, CT: Appleton & Lange, 1989:615.*)

Table 7-1
MUSCLES ACTING ON THE KNEE JOINT

	MUSCLES	INNERVATION
Extension	Quadriceps group: rectus femoris, vastus lateralis, interomedialis, and medialis	Femoral nerve
Flexion	Hamstring group: semitendinosus, semimembranosus, and biceps femoris	Tibial portion of sciatic nerve
Lateral rotation	Biceps femoris	Tibial portion of sciatic nerve
Medial rotation	Popliteus, semitendinosus, and semimembranosus	Tibial nerve

bursae (bursitis) will likely result in swelling of the entire knee joint. The knee joint is richly supplied by several **genicular and recurrent arteries from the femoral, popliteal, and anterior tibial arteries.**

Additional strength and stability to the knee joint are provided by the muscles that cross and produce movement at the joint. The action and innervation of these muscles are listed in Table 7-1.

An abnormal **force applied to the lateral aspect of the knee** with the foot planted **stretches the tibial (MCL) collateral ligament,** causing a sprain or, if forceful enough, rupture of this ligament. The exposed lateral knee makes this injury more frequent. Because the medial meniscus is firmly attached to the deep surface of the tibial collateral ligament, it also is frequently damaged. Forces applied to the medial aspect of the knee can damage the fibular (lateral) collateral ligament in a similar manner. However, because the lateral meniscus is not attached to the ligament, it typically is not damaged. Excessive force to the anterior aspect of the tibia will move it posteriorly, thus stretching or tearing the PCL. The **ACL** is most often damaged when forces or activities produce **hyperextension of the knee.**

COMPREHENSION QUESTIONS

[7.1]   Your patient has sustained an external force to the knee. Which of the
following ligaments has prevented abduction of the leg at the knee?

  A. Oblique popliteal
  B. Anterior cruciate
  C. Posterior cruciate
  D. Lateral collateral
  E. Medial collateral

[7.2]   In this same patient, which of the following ligaments prevented posterior displacement of the tibia on the femur?

    A. Oblique popliteal
    B. Anterior cruciate
    C. Posterior cruciate
    D. Lateral collateral
    E. Medial collateral

[7.3]   You have examined a patient and find there is weakness in the ability to flex the knee. This indicates a problem with which of the following nerves?

    A. Femoral nerve
    B. Tibial nerve
    C. Common fibular nerve
    D. Deep fibular nerve
    E. Superficial fibular nerve

Answers

[7.1]   **E.** Abduction of the leg at the knee is limited by the medial or tibial collateral ligament.

[7.2]   **C.** Posterior displacement of the tibia on the femur is limited by the PCL.

[7.3]   **B.** The muscles that flex the knee are innervated by the tibial portion of the sciatic nerve.

ANATOMY PEARLS

 The **anterior** cruciate ligament is so named because it is attached to the **anterior** aspect of the tibia and prevents **anterior** displacement of the tibia on the femur.

 The tibial collateral ligament is attached to the medial meniscus; thus, both are often injured by an abnormal force to the lateral knee.

 The ACL is injured most often by hyperextension of the knee.

REFERENCES

    Moore KL, Dalley AF. Clinically Oriented Anatomy, 5th ed. Baltimore, MD: Lippincott Williams & Wilkins, 2006:684–701.
    Netter FH. Atlas of Human Anatomy, 4th ed. Philadelphia, PA: Saunders, 2006: plates 507–10.
    Snell RS. Clinical Anatomy by Regions, 8th ed. Baltimore, MD: Lippincott Williams & Wilkins, 2008:629–33.

A 23-year-old female is seen on the postpartum floor the day after delivering a 9-pound baby boy. She is concerned about her right foot which has become numb and weak since delivering the baby. Walking has been difficult for her because her right foot tends to drop and her toes drag. When asked about her labor course, she reports that she had an epidural with satisfactory pain relief but a difficult and prolonged pushing stage of labor (3 hours) in stirrups. She denies any back pain or problems with the other leg. On exam, she has decreased sensation on the top of right foot and lateral side of the lower leg along with an inability to dorsiflex the right foot, resulting in a foot drop. Minimal peripheral edema is seen in both lower extremities.

◆ **What is the most likely diagnosis?**

◆ **What factors likely led to this condition?**

ANSWERS TO CASE 8: COMMON FIBULAR NERVE INJURY

Summary: A 23-year-old female postpartum day 1 with right foot weakness, numbness, and foot drop after a difficult vaginal delivery.

◆ **Most likely diagnosis:** Common fibular nerve injury (compression)

◆ **Factors leading to injury:** Prolonged compression of common fibular nerve by stirrups and flexion at the knee

CLINICAL CORRELATION

Compression of the common fibular nerve during labor is the most common postpartum nerve injury of the lower extremity. Compression of the common fibular nerve occurs from both the flexion of the knees and compression from stirrup on lateral aspect of knee. The common fibular nerve may also be injured during knee surgery, trauma, or prolong periods of compression (coma, deep sleep, lower extremity cast). Because of the epidural anesthesia, the patient likely felt no pain from the prolonged compression. Injury to the common fibular nerve causes numbness, weakness to the lower leg/foot, and foot drop (inability to dorsiflex foot). The majority of compression injuries after delivery are self-limiting and improve with supportive care. Proper positioning of the patient requires a good understanding of anatomy to avoid periods of prolonged nerve compression.

APPROACH TO LOWER LIMB

Objectives

1. Be able to describe the origin, course, muscles innervated, and distal cutaneous regions supplied by the sciatic nerve and its tibial and common fibular branches.
2. Be able to describe the origin, course, muscles innervated, and distal cutaneous regions supplied by the femoral and obturator nerves.

Definitions

Epidural: The space external to the spinal cord's dura mater; anesthetic agents are injected into this space for epidural anesthesia.
Nerve compression: Pressure on a nerve such that neural transmission is temporarily blocked.
Dorsiflexion: Decrease in the angle between the lower leg and foot, as with walking on one's heels; the opposite of plantarflexion, as standing on tip toe.

DISCUSSION

The **sciatic nerve** (L4-S3) is the largest nerve in the body, arising from the lumbosacral plexus. It exits the pelvis through the **greater sciatic foramen,** inferior to the piriformis muscle (see Figure 8-1). The sciatic nerve is actually two nerves, the **tibial (medial) and common fibula (lateral) nerves,** loosely bound together by connective tissue, The tibial nerve is derived from the anterior division of the anterior rami, while the common fibular is derived from the posterior division of the anterior rami. No muscles of the gluteal region are innervated by the sciatic nerve. It descends in the posterior compartment of the thigh where its **tibial nerve innervates all the muscles (hip extensors and knee flexors) of the posterior thigh** except the short head of the biceps femoris (innervated by the common fibular nerve). At approximately superior angle of the popliteal fossa, the tibial and common fibular portions separate.

The **common fibular nerve** passes laterally, superficially, and **courses around the neck of the fibula** subcutaneously **where it has risk of injury or compression (Figure 8-2).** It then divides into its superficial fibular nerve, which innervates the fibular muscles (evertors) of the lateral compartment of the leg, and the skin of the lateral leg and dorsum of the foot. The deep fibular nerve enters the anterior compartment of the leg, and innervates the muscles of this compartment (dorsiflexors), intrinsic dorsal foot muscles, and the skin between the great and second toe. **Severing the deep fibular nerve results in a foot drop.**

The **tibial nerve** descends through the popliteal fossa, and enters the posterior compartment of the leg to innervate the posterior compartment muscles (plantarflexors and invertors). It also gives off a medial sural branch which joins the communicating sural branch of the common fibular to form the **sural nerve** which is sensory to the posterior aspect of the leg and lateral foot. At the level of the posterior malleolus, the tibial nerve divides into the **lateral and medial plantar nerves** which innervate the intrinsic muscles and skin of the sole of the foot. **Severing the tibial nerve in the leg results in an inability to stand on tip toes.**

The **femoral nerve** (L2-4) arises from the lumbar plexus. Exits the abdomen posterior to the inguinal ligament, and lies lateral and outside the femoral sheath and its contents. It innervates the muscles (hip flexors and knee extensors) of the anterior compartment of the thigh, and the skin of the anterior thigh and medial leg. The **obturator nerve** (L2-4) exits the abdomen through the obturator canal, and enters the medial compartment of the thigh to innervate these muscles (adductors), and a patch of skin on the medial side of the thigh.

Figure 8-1. Innervation of the thigh. (*Reproduced with permission from Lindner HH. Clinical Anatomy. Norwalk, CT: Appleton & Lange, 1989:606.*)

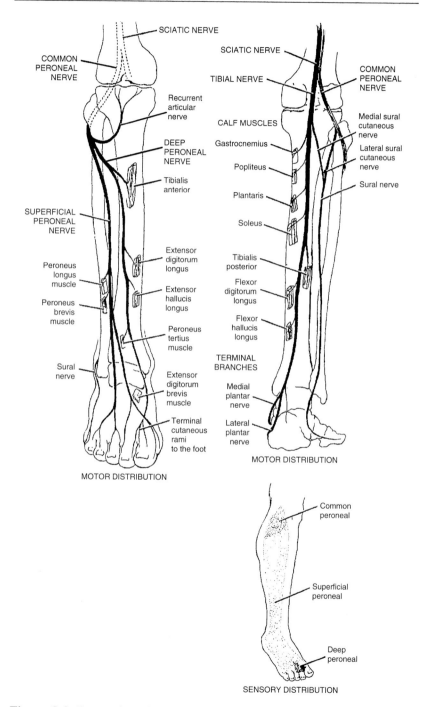

Figure 8-2. Innervation of the lower leg. (*Reproduced with permission from Lindner HH. Clinical Anatomy. Norwalk, CT: Appleton & Lange, 1989:50.*)

COMPREHENSION QUESTIONS

[8.1] During an abdominal hysterectomy for a cancerous uterus, the obturator nerve was accidentally severed. This resulted in the patient losing which of the following actions?

  A. Extension of the leg at the knee
  B. Extension of the thigh at the hip
  C. Adduction of the thigh at the hip
  D. Flexion of the leg at the knee
  E. Dorsiflexion of the foot at the ankle

[8.2] A patient comes to you complaining of his inability to stand on his tiptoes. Which of the following nerve injuries is most likely to be involved?

  A. Femoral nerve
  B. Tibial nerve
  C. Common fibular nerve
  D. Deep fibular nerve
  E. Superficial fibular nerve

[8.3] A 32-year-old woman is brought into the emergency department, because she is unable to evert her foot at the ankle. Which of the following nerve injuries is most likely to be involved?

  A. Femoral nerve
  B. Obturator nerve
  C. Tibial nerve
  D. Deep fibular nerve
  E. Superficial fibular nerve

Answers

[8.1] **C.** The obturator nerve innervates the muscles of the medial compartment of the thigh which adduct the thigh at the hip.

[8.2] **B.** The plantarflexors are located in the posterior compartment of the leg and innervated by the tibial nerve.

[8.3] **E.** The muscles of the lateral compartment of the leg evert the foot and are innervated by the superficial fibular nerve.

ANATOMY PEARLS

❖ The muscles of the posterior thigh, leg, and sole of the foot are all innervated by the tibial nerve (except the short head of the biceps femoris).

❖ The dorsiflexor muscles are innervated by the deep fibular nerve.

REFERENCES

Moore KL, Dalley AF. Clinically Oriented Anatpomy, 5th ed. Baltimore, MD: Lippincott Williams & Wilkins, 2006:597, 602, 621, 635, 642, 645, 655.

Netter FH. Atlas of Human Anatomy, 4th ed. Philadelphia, PA: Saunders, 2006: plates 538–42.

Snell RS. Clinical Anatomy by Regions, 8th ed. Baltimore, MD: Lippincott Williams & Wilkins, 2008:582, 586–7, 604, 614–5, 618.

❖ CASE 9

A 42-year-old diabetic woman complains of soreness of the left leg. She is moderately obese and has been recovering from surgical removal of her gall-bladder (cholecystectomy) performed 2 weeks ago. On examination, she has obvious swelling in the left lower leg and some tenderness of the calf that increases when the calf is gently squeezed. There is no redness of the leg, and she is afebrile (without fever).

◆ **What is the most likely diagnosis?**

◆ **What structure is likely affected?**

ANSWERS TO CASE 9: DEEP VENOUS THROMBOSIS

Summary: A 42-year-old obese diabetic woman complains of soreness of the left leg. She had gallbladder surgery 2 weeks previously. Her left calf is tender but without erythema. She is afebrile.

◆ **Most likely diagnosis:** Deep venous thrombosis (DVT)

◆ **Structure likely affected:** Anterior and posterior tibial veins and fibular veins

CLINICAL CORRELATION

Venous thrombosis, or pathological blood clots within a vein, is a common cause of morbidity and mortality. Virchow triad of venous stasis, hypercoagulability, and vessel wall damage comprises notable risk factors. This patient has several risk factors for DVT. She is obese, diabetic, and has been inactive due to postoperative bed rest, with the latter producing venous stasis. Although gynecological and orthopedic surgeries especially predispose to DVT, any surgery increases the risk. Prevention of DVT includes using lower limb compression devices during and after surgery. These devices intermittently "squeeze" the legs, thereby simulating the muscular contraction of physical activity. Anticoagulant therapy, such as small-dose heparin, is also sometimes given before surgery and for 1–2 days postoperatively. If DVT is confirmed with ultrasound or radiologically with venous contrast (venogram), anticoagulation therapy is important to decrease the risk of embolization of the thrombosis, which can travel directly to the lungs to produce potentially fatal pulmonary embolism.

APPROACH TO VASCULAR SUPPLY OF LOWER EXTREMITY

Objectives

1 Be able to draw the arterial blood supply to the lower limb.
2. Be able to describe the deep and superficial venous drainage of the lower limb.

Definitions

Afebrile: Without fever.
Embolus: A mass such as part of the blood clot (thrombus), air, or fat that travels through a vessel and lodges and obstructs the blood flow.
Thrombosis: Process by which a blood clot forms within a blood vessel.

DISCUSSION

The **chief blood supply to the lower limb is from the femoral artery,** the continuation of the **external iliac artery** inferior to the inguinal ligament, within the **femoral triangle.** The **femoral triangle** is bounded by the **inguinal ligament superiorly,** the **sartorius muscle laterally,** and the **adductor longus muscle medially.** It contains the femoral nerve and the femoral sheath and its contents. The femoral artery lies in the lateral compartment of the **femoral sheath,** with the **femoral vein** medial to it, and the femoral canal with its associated inguinal lymph nodes medial to the vein. The femoral nerve lies lateral to and outside the femoral sheath. Just inferior to the inguinal ligament, the **superficial epigastric, superficial circumflex iliac,** and **two external pudendal arteries arise from the femoral artery.** Within the **femoral triangle,** the deep femoral artery arises and descends posteriorly to the femoral vessels and the adductor longus muscle. The **lateral and medial circumflex arteries** usually arise from the **deep femoral artery,** as do muscular branches and several perforating branches, to supply the posterior thigh. As the femoral artery descends toward the apex of the femoral triangle, it enters the **adductor canal** and becomes the **popliteal artery,** and it assumes a position posterior to the femur. It descends inferiorly through the popliteal fossa, giving rise to five genicular arteries to the knee, and terminates by dividing into the **anterior and posterior tibial arteries** near the lower border of the popliteus muscle (Figure 9-1).

The **anterior tibial artery** pierces the **interosseus membrane** from which it descends through the **anterior compartment,** supplying structures in this compartment, and terminates anterior to the ankle by becoming the **dorsal artery of the foot.** The dorsal artery and its lateral tarsal branch form an **arch of the dorsum of the foot** and is the chief blood supply to the toes. The **posterior tibial artery** descends in the posterior compartment and supplies it and the lateral compartment by perforating branches in addition to its fibular branch. It passes posteriorly to the **medial malleolus,** enters the sole of the foot, and divides into lateral and medial plantar arteries that supply the sole of the foot.

Other arteries that supply portions of the lower limb include the **obturator artery,** which supplies the medial compartment of the thigh. The **superior and inferior gluteal and the internal pudendal arteries** provide the chief blood supply to the gluteal region.

The lower limb has **superficial and deep systems of veins,** both of which terminate in the **femoral vein,** which continues superiorly to the inguinal ligament as the external iliac vein. The deep system of veins usually consists of **paired venae comitantes,** which accompany the arteries for which they are named. Thus anterior and posterior tibial veins are formed from the dorsum and sole of the foot. Fibular veins arise in the posterior compartment and drain blood to the posterior tibial veins, which ascend and are joined by the anterior tibial veins to form the popliteal vein. The **popliteal vein** becomes the **femoral vein** as it traverses the **adductor canal,** receives the deep femoral vein in the femoral sheath, and enters the abdomen beneath the inguinal canal to become

Figure 9-1. Arterial supply to the leg. (*Reproduced, with permission, from Lindner HH. Clinical Anatomy. East Norwalk, CT: Appleton & Lange, 1989:602.*)

the external iliac vein. A deep vein of the thigh accompanies its artery and drains into the femoral. The superficial system of veins is composed of the **small and great saphenous veins** and are found in the superficial fascial of the limb. The small saphenous is formed posterior to the lateral malleolus and ascends in the middle of the calf to terminate in the popliteal vein in the popliteal fossa. The **great saphenous is formed from the dorsal venous arch**

of the foot anterior to the medial malleolus. It ascends along the **medial aspect of the leg and thigh.** It pierces the saphenous opening in the fascia lata (deep fascia of the thigh) to empty into the femoral vein within the femoral sheath. Numerous communications exist between the two saphenous veins. Of greater clinical importance, **communications between the superficial and deep systems exist as perforating branches,** whose valves are arranged to allow venous flow from superficial to deep, but not in the opposite direction. This important shunt allows muscular contraction to produce venous return against the effects of gravity.

COMPREHENSION QUESTIONS

[9.1]   As an orthopedic surgeon is operating in the posterior compartment of the thigh, care is taken to preserve the arterial blood supply to the muscles in that region. These are branches of which of the following arteries?

A. Deep femoral artery
B. Femoral artery
C. Superior gluteal artery
D. Inferior gluteal artery
E. Obturator artery

[9.2]   A patient has sustained lower limb trauma that has damaged the posterior tibial artery. Therefore, you will be concerned about the blood supply to which of the following?

A. Posterior thigh only
B. Lateral compartment of the leg only
C. Posterior compartment of the leg only
D. Sole of the foot only
E. Posterior compartment of the leg and the sole of the foot

[9.3]   Which are the chief deep veins of the leg that are of concern for DVT?

A. Small saphenous vein
B. Great saphenous vein
C. Deep femoral vein
D. Anterior and posterior tibial veins
E. Obturator vein

Answers

[9.1]   **A.** The blood supply to the posterior compartment of the thigh is from perforating branches of the deep femoral artery.

[9.2]   **E.** The posterior tibial artery provides the blood supply to the calf and sole of the foot.

[9.3]   **D.** The deep veins of the leg are the anterior and posterior tibial veins that accompany the arteries of the same name.

ANATOMY PEARLS

 The relation of lateral to medial of structures within the femoral triangle is defined by the mnemonic NAVeL (femoral Nerve, Artery, Vein; empty space, Lymph nodes).

 The chief blood supply to the thigh and hip arises from the deep femoral artery.

 The posterior tibial artery enters the foot through the tarsal canal, posterior to the medial malleolus.

 Venous blood flow is from superficial to deep venous systems.

REFERENCES

Moore KL, Dalley AF. Clinically Oriented Anatomy, 5th ed. Baltimore, MD: Lippincott Williams & Wilkins, 2006:580–4. 603–6, 655–6.

Netter FH. Atlas of Human Anatomy, 4th ed. Philadelphia, PA: Saunders, 2006: plates 500, 512, 518.

Snell RS. Clinical Anatomy by Regions, 8th ed. Baltimore, MD: Lippincott Williams & Wilkins, 2008:570–2, 580–2, 617–8.

A 42-year-old man is brought to the emergency room complaining of intense pain in his left calf and ankle. He had entered a tennis tournament with his 15-year-old son and states that, as he lunged after a hard-hit serve, he heard a "snap," fell to the court in tremendous pain, and could not walk. On examination, the left calf is tender and indurated, with an irregular mass noted in the back of the midcalf area.

◆ **What is the most likely diagnosis?**

◆ **What type of excessive abnormal ankle movement would be present?**

ANSWERS TO CASE 10: ACHILLES TENDON RUPTURE

Summary: A 42-year-old man heard a "snap" while playing tennis and experienced left calf pain after lunging for a ball. The left calf is tender and indurated and has a lump.

◆ **Most likely diagnosis:** Achilles tendon rupture

◆ **Likely abnormal ankle movement present:** Dorsiflexion

CLINICAL CORRELATION

The gastrocnemius and soleus muscles form a three-headed muscle group (triceps surae) that unite to form a single tendon, the calcaneal or Achilles tendon, which inserts into the calcaneus bone. These muscles produce plantar flexion of the foot at the ankle and limit dorsiflexion. Running or quick-start athletic activity, such as described in this case, may lead to strain or rupture of the tendon. The snap heard by this patient is fairly common in calcaneal tendon avulsion. The mass noted in the left calf is due to foreshortening of the triceps surae. Compared with the opposite side, the affected foot will have greater range of motion in dorsiflexion and loss of plantar flexion. Treatment is usually surgical repair of the tendon. Due to the limited blood supply to this tendon, a long immobilization is typically required. Postoperative physical therapy to prevent tendon contracture is critical.

APPROACH TO THE ANKLE JOINT

Objectives

1. Be able to describe the anatomy of the ankle joint.
2. Be able to describe the muscles that cross the ankle joint, the movements they produce, and the ligaments that limit these movements.

Definitions

Indurated: Process in which usually soft tissue becomes extremely hard.
Strain: Injury that results from overuse or inappropriate use.
Avulsion: Violent separation or tearing away.

DISCUSSION

Movements of the foot at the ankle occur at two joints: the **ankle joint proper** or **talocrural joint,** which is formed by the distal ends or malleoli of the fibula and tibia, and the trochlea of the talus bone. A **mortise-shaped joint** is formed at which the hinged movements of **dorsi- and plantarflexion** occur. The ankle

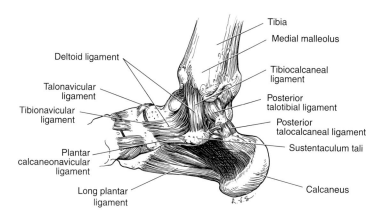

Figure 10-1. The medial ligaments of the ankle joint. (*Reproduced, with permission, from Lindner HH. Clinical Anatomy. East Norwalk, CT:Appleton & Lange, 1989:638.*)

joint is more stable in dorsiflexion because the anterior aspect of the trochlea is tightly wedged between the lateral and medial malleoli. The movements of **inversion and eversion** of the foot occur primarily at the **subtalar joint** (between the talus and calcaneus bones), but also at the transverse tarsal joint with articulation of the talus and calcaneus bones with the navicular and cuboid bones (Figures 10-1 and 10-2).

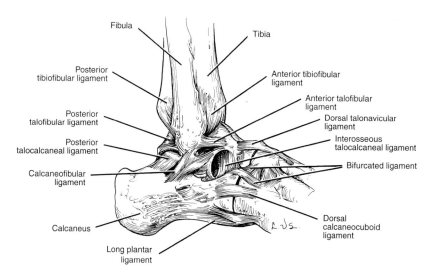

Figure 10-2. The lateral ligaments of the ankle joint. (*Reproduced, with permission, from Lindner HH. Clinical Anatomy. East Norwalk, CT:Appleton & Lange, 1989:639.*)

Table 10-1
MUSCLES ACTING ON THE FOOT

	MUSCLE	INNERVATION
Dorsiflexion	Tibialis anterior, extensor digitorum longus, extensor hallucis longus, fibularis tertius	Deep fibular nerve
Plantarflexion	Triceps surae: gastrocnemius, soleus, plantaris; flexor hallucis longus, flexor digitorum longus, tibialis posterior	Tibial nerve
Inversion	Tibialis anterior	Deep fibular nerve
	Tibialis posterior	Tibial nerve
Eversion	Fibularis longus, and brevis	Superficial fibular nerve
	Fibularis tertius	Deep fibular nerve

The capsule of the ankle joint is thin anteriorly and posteriorly, but ligaments reinforce the capsule laterally and medially to provide much of the stability. A **relatively weak lateral ligament** is formed by **three individual ligaments,** all of which attach to the lateral malleolus of the fibula: anterior and posterior talofibular ligaments and calcaneofibular ligaments. The **lateral ligament limits excessive inversion.** The medial (deltoid) ligament is a very strong ligament composed of four individual ligaments that attach to the tibia: tibionavicular, anterior and posterior tibiotalar, and tibiocalcaneal ligaments. The **medial ligament limits eversion.** The muscles that produce dorsiflexion at the ankle are located in the anterior compartment of the leg, whereas the muscles that cause plantar flexion and eversion are located in the posterior and lateral compartments, respectively. The muscles that produce movements of the foot at the ankle are listed in Table 10-1.

COMPREHENSION QUESTIONS

[10.1] When will a patient's ankle joint have the greatest stability?

    A. When the knee is flexed
    B. When the foot is dorsiflexed
    C. When the foot is plantarflexed
    D. When the foot is everted
    E. When the foot is inverted

[10.2] You are concerned that your patient's medial deltoid ligament may have been torn from its proximal attachment. Which of the following would you palpate for tenderness?

A. The medial aspect of the tibial shaft
B. The lateral aspect of the fibular shaft
C. The lateral malleolus
D. The medial malleolus
E. The calcaneus

[10.3] Your female patient is unable to walk on her tiptoes. You immediately suspect damage to which of the following nerves?

A. Sural nerve
B. Tibial nerve
C. Common fibular nerve
D. Superficial fibular nerve
E. Deep fibular nerve

Answers

[10.1] **B.** The talocrural or ankle joint proper has the greatest stability in dorsiflexion.

[10.2] **D.** The four components of the deltoid ligament arise from the medial malleolus.

[10.3] **B.** Plantarflexion of the foot at the ankle is produced by the muscles in the calf, which are innervated by the tibial nerve.

ANATOMY PEARLS

 Dorsiflexion and plantarflexion occur at the ankle joint proper, whereas inversion and eversion occur primarily at the subtalar joint.
 A patient with a lesion of the tibial nerve above the knee would be unable to stand on tiptoes (plantarflex the foot at the ankle).
 A patient with foot drop and inability to evert the foot (walk on the instep) has a lesion of the common fibular nerve (which is at risk as it passes around the neck of the fibula).

REFERENCES

Moore KL, Dalley AF. Clinically Oriented Anatomy, 5th ed. Baltimore, MD: Lippincott Williams & Wilkins, 2006:647–52, 702–7.
Netter FH. Atlas of Human Anatomy, 4th ed. Philadelphia, PA: Saunders, 2006: plates 517, 521, 527.
Snell RS. Clinical Anatomy by Regions, 8th ed. Baltimore, MD: Lippincott Williams & Wilkins, 2008:615–7, 634–6.

A 48-year-old man complains of swelling of the neck and shortness of breath of 1-week duration. He has noticed some nasal stuffiness with hoarseness of his voice for about 3 weeks and had attributed these symptoms to an upper respiratory infection. He denies the use of alcohol but has smoked two packs of cigarettes per day for 30 years. Lately, he feels as though something is pushing against his throat. On physical examination, the patient's face appears ruddy and swollen. The jugular veins are distended.

◆ **What is the most likely diagnosis?**

◆ **What is the most likely cause?**

◆ **What are the anatomical structures involved?**

ANSWERS TO CASE 11: SUPERIOR VENA CAVA SYNDROME

Summary: A 48-year-old heavy smoker has a 1-week history of neck swelling, dyspnea, and the sensation of something pushing on his throat. Three weeks ago, he developed nasal stuffiness and voice hoarseness. He has facial plethora, edema, and jugular venous distention.

◆ **Most likely diagnosis:** Superior vena cava (SVC) syndrome

◆ **Most likely cause:** Bronchogenic lung cancer

◆ **Anatomical structures likely involved:** SVC, trachea, and right mainstem bronchus

CLINICAL CORRELATION

The SVC receives venous drainage from the head, neck, upper limb, and thorax. Located in the upper mediastinum, this thin-walled vessel is susceptible to pressure from external sources. The most common cause of such external compression is malignancy, usually from a right-side bronchogenic carcinoma. Such tumors can also compress the trachea, producing dyspnea, and may involve the recurrent laryngeal nerve, producing hoarseness, as in this patient. The stellate sympathetic ganglion may be compressed, leading to a Horner syndrome, the clinical triad of unilateral miosis (constricted pupil), facial anhydrosis (dryness), and ptosis (drooping eyelid). The development of SVC syndrome is often an emergency because the trachea may be obstructed, leading to respiratory compromise. The priority in treatment is directed toward the airway, with oxygen and possibly diuretic agents, and corticosteroid agents to relieve the edema. A chest radiograph, computed tomographic (CT) scan, and a tissue biopsy, in that order, would be the next diagnostic steps. Most patients who have lung cancer are treated with radiotherapy. Although patients who have SVC syndrome often respond well to the radiation treatment, the overall prognosis is nearly always poor due to the advanced extent of the cancer.

APPROACH TO THE MEDIASTINUM

Objectives

1. Be able to describe the divisions of the mediastinum and the contents of each.
2. Be able to describe the lymphatic drainage of the thoracic organs.

Definitions

Superior vena cava syndrome: Engorgement of the vessels of the head, neck, and upper limbs accompanied by cough and respiratory difficulty due to compression of the SVC or its main tributaries by a benign or malignant mass.

Bronchogenic carcinoma: A malignant tumor arising from the mucosal epithelium of the large bronchi.

Mediastinum: The central region of the thorax between the two pleural cavities.

DISCUSSION

The **mediastinum** is the central portion of the thoracic cavity, and it lies between the two pulmonary cavities. It is bounded laterally by the mediastinal pleura. It contains all the thoracic viscera except the two lungs. **Superior and inferior divisions** are described, with the latter further divided into **anterior, middle, and posterior divisions.**

The **superior mediastinum** extends from the superior thoracic aperture bounded by the superior border of the manubrium, first rib, and T1 vertebral body. The inferior boundary is a horizontal line from the sternal angle posterior to the intervertebral disc between T4 and T5. The superior mediastinum contains the following structures, from anterior to posterior: adipose tissue with remnants of the thymus gland, right and left brachiocephalic vein, SVC, aorta with its brachiocephalic trunk, left common carotid and left subclavian arterial branches, trachea, esophagus, and thoracic duct. Related to these structures are the phrenic, vagus, left recurrent laryngeal and cardiac nerves, and anterior mediastinal lymph node group (Figure 11-1).

The **inferior mediastinum** is bounded anteriorly by the sternum, posteriorly by vertebral bodies T5 through T12, and the diaphragm inferiorly. The **anterior mediastinum** portion lies between the sternum and the pericardial sac and contains small branches of the internal thoracic artery and a few nodes of the parasternal lymph node group. The thymus gland is present during childhood. The **middle mediastinum** contains the pericardial sac with the heart, terminations of the SVC, inferior vena cava (IVC), and pulmonary veins, the ascending aorta, the pulmonary trunk and its bifurcations into the right and left pulmonary arteries, lung roots, phrenic nerve, and bronchial lymph nodes. The **posterior mediastinum** lies between the pericardial sac and vertebral bodies T5 through T12. It contains the esophagus, descending thoracic aorta and right intercostals and esophageal arteries, azygous venous system, thoracic duct, vagus and splanchnic nerves, and posterior mediastinal lymph nodes.

The body's main lymphatic vessel, the **thoracic duct,** originates in the abdomen at the level of L1 as a highly variable dilation called the **cisterna chili.** It enters the posterior mediastinum through the aortic hiatus and lies on the right anterior surface of the thoracic vertebral bodies, posterior to the

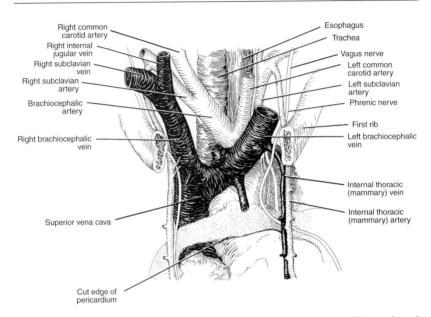

Figure 11-1. The superior mediastinum and root of the neck. (*Reproduced, with permission, from Lindner HH. Clinical Anatomy. East Norwalk, CT: Appleton & Lange, 1989:226.*)

esophagus between the **azygous venous system** and the thoracic aorta. By the level of the sternal angle, the duct completes a shift to the left side, traverses the superior mediastinum, and terminates by emptying into the venous system near the junction of the left internal jugular and subclavian veins. The **thoracic duct receives lymph drainage from the lower limbs, abdomen and left hemithorax, upper limb, and head and neck.** A small right lymphatic duct receives lymph drainage from the right hemithorax, upper limb, and head and neck. The thoracic and right lymphatic ducts are described as receiving lymph from jugular, subclavian, and bronchomediastinal trunks, although these trunks may variably unite or empty into veins independently.

Lymph node groups that drain lymph from the thoracic wall include the parasternal, intercostals, and several diaphragmatic groups. Lymph nodes that drain thoracic viscera include anterior mediastinal nodes in the anterior region of the superior mediastinum and those located on the anterior surfaces of the brachiocephalic veins, SVC, and the aortic arch and its branches. These nodes receive lymph from the thymus, inferior part of the thyroid gland, heart, pericardium, mediastinal pleura, lung hilum, and parasternal and diaphragmatic nodes. Vessels from the anterior mediastinal help form the right and left bronchomediastinal trunks. Posterior mediastinal nodes lie along the esophagus and thoracic aorta and drain lymph from the esophagus, pericardium, diaphragm, and superior surface of the liver. The vessels from this group empty into the thoracic duct or tracheobronchial nodes (Figure 11-2).

The largest number of visceral nodes are associated with the lungs and airways. The lungs have **superficial and deep lymphatic plexuses** that drain into the bronchopulmonary (hilar) lymph node. The **deep plexuses,** however,

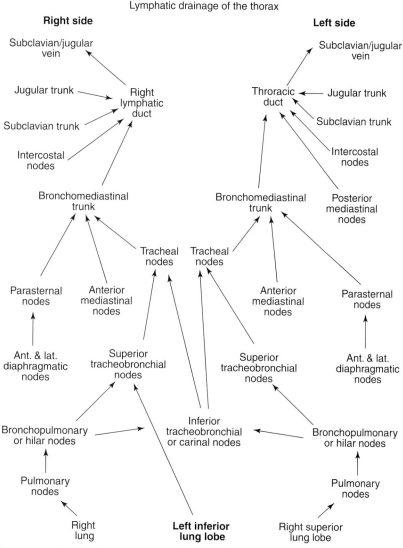

Note: The jugular, subclavian and bronchomediastinal trunks may empty into the right lymphatic and thoracic ducts as illustrated here, or directly into the venous system.

Figure 11-2. Lymphatic flow through the chest.

first drain through pulmonary nodes along the bronchi within the lung, from which the lymph passes to the bronchopulmonary nodes. Lymph then drains to **inferior and superior tracheobronchial nodes** (below and above the tracheal bifurcation) and **tracheal nodes** located along the sides of the trachea. The tracheobronchial nodes on the right side are closely related to the SVC and receive lymph from the right lung and the inferior part of the left lung. Vessels from these node groups form the right and left bronchomediastinal trunks.

COMPREHENSION QUESTIONS

[11.1] A thoracic surgeon has entered the right pleural cavity and excised two suspicious lymph nodes at the hilum of the right lung for frozen-section pathological study. These nodes belong to which of the following lymph node groups?

    A. Parasternal
    B. Paratracheal
    C. Superior tracheobronchial
    D. Inferior tracheobronchial
    E. Bronchopulmonary

[11.2] During a surgical procedure, a surgeon has reflected the fat pad containing the thymic remnants and notes a large venous structure crossing the midline from the left and apparently emptying into the SVC. This vessel is most likely which of the following?

    A. Right brachiocephalic vein
    B. Left brachiocephalic vein
    C. Left internal jugular vein
    D. Left subclavian vein
    E. Azygous vein

[11.3] A pediatric heart surgeon has just divided the sternum in a child to repair a cardiac malformation. A lobulated gland-like structure is seen immediately obscuring the heart. This is most likely which of the following?

    A. Lung
    B. Thyroid gland
    C. Thymus
    D. Lymph nodes
    E. Liver

Answers

[11.1]   **E.** The bronchopulmonary lymph node group is located at the hilum of each lung, and it receives lymph from the superficial and deep lymphatic plexuses.

[11.2]   **B.** The left brachiocephalic vein crosses the midline to unite with the almost vertical right brachiocephalic vein to form the SVC.

[11.3]   **C.** The anterior mediastinum lies immediately posterior to the sternum and contains the thymus in children.

ANATOMY PEARLS

 The surface landmark for the boundary between the superior and inferior (anterior, middle, and posterior) mediastinum is the sternal angle.

 The thoracic duct is found in the posterior and superior mediastina.

 The right tracheobronchial nodes drain lymph from the right lung and inferior portion of the left lung.

 Much of the lymph from the thorax and its contents will drain into the bronchomediastinal trunk.

REFERENCES

Clemente CD, ed. Gray's Anatomy of the Human Body, 30th American ed. Philadelphia, PA: Lea & Febiger, 1985:890–6.

Moore KL, Dalley AF. Clinically Oriented Anatomy, 5th ed. Baltimore, MD: Lippincott Williams & Wilkins, 2006:130–2, 135–7, 169–75.

Netter FH. Atlas of Human Anatomy, 4th ed. Philadelphia, PA: Saunders, 2006: plates 206, 208.

❖ CASE 12

A 60-year-old woman is noted to have a 2-cm mass in the left breast. The patient's physician recommends that a core needle biopsy be performed. Tissue analysis by the pathologist under the microscope reveals intraductal carcinoma. The patient is advised by the surgeon to have surgery to remove the primary breast mass in addition to some lymph nodes. The patient undergoes wide excision of the breast mass and lymph node removal.

◆ **Which lymph nodes are most likely to be affected?**

◆ **What anatomical structure defines the "levels" of lymph nodes?**

ANSWERS TO CASE 12: BREAST CANCER

Summary: A 60-year-old woman undergoes lumpectomy and lymph node dissection for a 2-cm intraductal carcinoma of the breast.

◆ **Most likely lymph nodes affected:** Axillary nodes.

◆ **Anatomical structure that defines the "levels" of lymph nodes:** The pectoralis minor muscle is used to define lymph node levels. Levels 1, 2, and 3 are lateral to, deep to, and medial to the pectoralis minor, respectively.

CLINICAL CORRELATION

This 60-year-old woman had a palpable breast mass. Pathological examination revealed intraductal carcinoma in the core needle biopsy. Risk factors include the patient's age, and intraductal carcinoma is the most common histological type. The most common treatment plan would be a breast-conserving procedure such as a lumpectomy (excising the malignant mass with some margins) and axillary lymph node dissection. The presence or absence of malignant cells in the axillary lymph nodes is the single most important prognostic factor for survival. **Options for nodal staging include level 1 and 2 axillary node dissection versus sentinel node biopsy.** The sentinel node(s) represents the node(s) to which primary lymph drainage occurs from a tumor or anatomical site. It is identified by injection of radiotracers and a blue dye at the primary tumor site. Biopsy of the sentinel node(s) results in a smaller incision and decreased trauma to the axilla. However, if the sentinel node(s) is positive for metastatic disease, a complete level 1 and 2 axillary dissection should be performed.

Other physical signs of breast cancer, which this patient did not have, include skin dimpling or retraction, which is formed by the underlying cancer adherent to the fibrous septa of the breast, or the thickened red appearance of *peau d'orange,* which is caused by the malignant cells proliferating within the lymphatics underlying the skin. A red warm breast in a non–breast-feeding woman can also represent inflammatory breast cancer due to malignancy within the lymphatic channels of the skin.

APPROACH TO THE AXILLARY LYMPH NODES

Objectives

1. Be able to describe the anatomy of the adult female breast, including the blood and nerve supplies.
2. Be able to list the primary path for lymphatic drainage of the breast and the several subgroups of the axillary nodes.
3. Be able to describe the secondary pathways for lymph drainage.

Definitions

Axilla: Small pyramidal space between the upper lateral chest and the medial arm, including the blood vessels, nerves, and lymph nodes.

Tail of Spence: A protrusion of mammary tissue into the axilla that sometimes enlarges premenstrually.

Axillary lymph node dissection: Surgical excision of lymph nodes of the axilla usually related to breast cancer for diagnostic and therapeutic reasons.

Peau d'orange: Orange peel appearance of the skin of the breast with edema and prominent pores secondary to obstruction of lymphatics by a tumor with associated inflammation.

DISCUSSION

The adult female breast consists of subcutaneous, radially arranged, mammary gland tissue and fat, typically extending from ribs 2 through 6 superiorly to inferiorly and from the sternal border to the midaxillary line (Figure 12-1). The **long thoracic nerve** lies close to the midaxillary line. For descriptive purposes, it is divided into quadrants. Each breast is centered by the elevated nipple, which contains the openings of the **lactiferous ducts** and is composed of circular smooth muscle. Surrounding the nipple is pigmented skin or the areola, which contains the opening of the lubricating sebaceous glands. The radially arranged mammary gland tissue forms **15 to 20 lobes,** each drained by a lactiferous duct that has a dilatation called the **lactiferous sinus** just before its opening onto the nipple. The lobes are irregularly separated by incomplete dense connective tissue septae that attach to the dermis of the overlying skin. These **septae, called the suspensory ligaments (of Cooper),** are especially well developed in the superior half of the breast. A loose connective tissue layer, the retromammary space, separates the breast components and the **pectoral fascia,** allowing for some movement. The breast overlies the pectoralis major and the anterior portion of the serratus anterior muscles. A portion of breast tissue typically extends into the axilla as the **axillary tail (of Spence).** The breast is supplied by branches of the **internal thoracic, lateral thoracic, and anterior and posterior intercostal arteries. The breast is innervated by anterior and lateral cutaneous branches of intercostal nerves.**

  Lymphatic drainage of the breast begins as a subareolar plexus. The majority of lymph drained from the breast (usually quantified at 75%) **drains to the axillary lymph nodes.** The axillary node group is often described as a pyramid, like the axilla, and is typically subdivided into **five subgroups: pectoral (anterior), lateral (humeral), posterior (subscapular), central (medial), and apical.** Lymph from the axillary nodes typically drains into the **inferior deep cervical lymph nodes.** However, lymph from the axillary node group may drain into other nodes such as the interpectoral and deltopectoral nodes

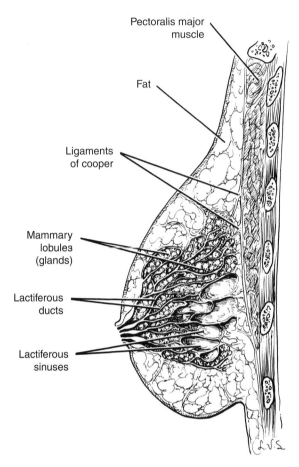

Figure 12-1. Saggital section of the breast. (*Reproduced, with permission, from Lindner HH. Clinical Anatomy. East Norwalk, CT: Appleton & Lange, 1989:202.*)

(Figure 12-2). This is especially true in instances of metastasis because "normal" paths become blocked by the malignancy and alternate routes must be established. **The pectoral, humeral, and subscapular nodes are level 1 nodes, whereas the central and apical nodes are level 2 and 3 nodes, respectively.**

The **medial quadrants of the breast will have lymph drain into the parasternal lymph nodes** along the **internal thoracic vessels.** Some lymph from the inferior quadrants may drain to **inferior phrenic nodes.**

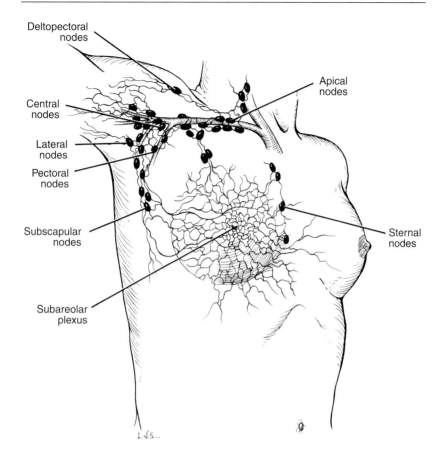

Figure 12-2. Lymphatics of the breast. (*Reproduced, with permission, from Lindner HH. Clinical Anatomy. East Norwalk, CT: Appleton & Lange, 1989:205.*)

COMPREHENSION QUESTIONS

[12.1] A 45-year-old woman is noted to have a 1.5-cm breast cancer located in the upper inner quadrant of the right breast. Which of the following lymph nodes is most likely to be affected?

A. Level 1 axillary node
B. Level 2 axillary node
C. Level 3 axially node
D. Parasternal node
E. Inferior phrenic node

[12.2] A physician is performing a breast examination. In addition to the breast tissue on the chest, what other region is critical to complete the palpation of mammary tissue?

A. Supraclavicular region
B. Subclavicular region
C. Axillary region
D. Parasternal region

[12.3] A 24-year-old woman has vaginally delivered an infant 2 days ago. She complains of breast engorgement and swelling in regions at about the level of the umbilicus and at the lateral abdomen. There seems to be some leaking from these areas of swelling. Which of the following is the most likely diagnosis?

A. Bilateral lipoma
B. Accessory breast tissue
C. Ascites
D. Cutaneous malignancy

Answers

[12.1]   **D.** Cancers located in the medial breast usually drain to the parasternal nodes.

[12.2]   **C.** The tail of Spence is located in the axillary area and contains mammary tissue.

[12.3]   **B.** These areas likely are accessory breast tissue. The "milk line" extends from the axilla to the groin area, and accessory mammary tissue may be present anywhere along this line.

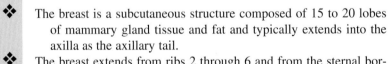

ANATOMY PEARLS

❖ The breast is a subcutaneous structure composed of 15 to 20 lobes of mammary gland tissue and fat and typically extends into the axilla as the axillary tail.

❖ The breast extends from ribs 2 through 6 and from the sternal border to the midaxillary line. This places the lateral thoracic nerve at risk during surgery.

❖ The suspensory ligaments of the breast are attached to the dermis of the skin.

❖ The majority of lymph from the breast drains to the axillary lymph nodes, with secondary drainage to the parasternal and inferior phrenic nodes.

REFERENCES

Moore KL, Dalley AF. Clinically Oriented Anatomy, 5th ed. Baltimore, MD: Lippincott Williams & Wilkins, 2006:105–12.

Netter FH. Atlas of Human Anatomy, 4th ed. Philadelphia, PA: Saunders, 2006 plates 182–4.

Snell RS. Clinical Anatomy by Regions, 8th ed. Baltimore, MD: Lippincott Williams & Wilkins, 2008:427–32.

A 35-year-old Hispanic woman comes to your office tired and complaining of shortness of breath and fatigue. Her history is unremarkable except for a vague history of fever and joint pain as a child in Mexico. She notes some recent fatigue and difficulty sleeping that she attributes to job stress. On examination, her heart rate is 120 beats/min, and the rhythm has no discernible pattern (irregularly irregular). Auscultation of the heart indicates a systolic murmur (during left ventricular ejection of blood) that is harsh in character.

◆ **What is the most likely diagnosis?**

◆ **What is the underlying etiology?**

ANSWERS TO CASE 13: ATRIAL FIBRILLATION/ MITRAL STENOSIS

Summary: A 35-year-old Hispanic woman complains of fatigue. She had fever and joint pain as a child in Mexico. On examination, her heart rate is 120 beats/min and irregularly irregular. Cardiac examination shows a harsh systolic murmur.

◆   **Most likely diagnosis:** Atrial fibrillation due to left atrial enlargement

◆   **Underlying etiology:** Mitral stenosis due to rheumatic heart disease

CLINICAL CORRELATION

This 35-year-old woman most likely has atrial fibrillation with tachycardia that is irregularly irregular. Instead of the electrical impulse originating from the sinoatrial (SA) node of the right atrium and depolarizing both atria in a regular, orderly manner, this patient's atria have constant electrical stimulation, leading to almost continual atrial contraction that visually resembles a "bag of worms." The irregular character of the pulse is the result of inconsistent transmission of the electrical impulse to and through the atrioventricular (AV) node and then onto the two ventricles. One common cause of atrial fibrillation is left atrial enlargement. In this patient, the history of childhood fever and joint pain likely is the result of streptococcally caused rheumatic fever. If untreated, the microorganism can cause inflammation of the mitral valve, leading to mitral stenosis. Over the course of years, the mitral stenosis is likely to worsen, leading to atrial enlargement, fibrillation, and pulmonary edema with intolerance to physical exertion. Treatment in this patient would focus on decreasing her heart rate with an agent that acts on the AV node such as digoxin. Oxygen and diuretics would relieve her pulmonary symptoms. An ultimate goal will be the conversion of her cardiac contractions to a normal sinus rhythm. Anticoagulation is often warranted in the face of long-term atrial fibrillation because of the likelihood of intracardiac thrombus and the possibility of emboli after conversion to sinus rhythm, called the "atrial stunning" effect. Surgical correction of the mitral stenosis is also important.

APPROACH TO CARDIAC CONDUCTION SYSTEM

Objectives

1. Be able to describe the type of tissue that makes up the cardiac conduction system.
2. Be able to describe the locations and functions of the SA node, AV node, bundle, and the right and left bundle branches.
3. Be able to describe the nature of sinus rhythm and the influence of the divisions of the autonomic nervous system on this rhythm.
4. Be able to describe the anatomy of the four cardiac valves.

Definitions

Murmurs: Soft or harsh abnormal heart sounds, often caused by turbulent blood flow, and described in relation to the phase of the cardiac cycle in which they are heard.

Atrial fibrillation: Rapid, uncoordinated muscular twitching of the atrial wall.

Tachycardia: A heart rate of at least 100 beats/min.

DISCUSSION

Cardiac Conduction System

The conduction system of the heart is composed of specially modified cardiac muscle cells. It initiates and rapidly conducts cardiac impulses throughout the heart to produce cardiac muscle contraction. The system ensures the simultaneous contraction of both atria, followed by a similar coordinated contraction of both ventricles.

The **SA node,** composed of these modified cardiac muscle cells, lies within the **atrial wall on the right side** of its junction with the **SVC.** This can be located at the superior end of the external landmark, the **sulcus terminalis.** The SA node spontaneously depolarizes to initiate the cardiac conduction impulse and thus is often referred to as the **heart's pacemaker.** The impulse generated by the SA node spreads through the atrial wall to converge on the **AV node** and produces simultaneous atrial contraction. **Anterior, middle, and posterior internodal pathways** of very rapid conduction are described (Figure 13-1).

The **AV node** is a somewhat smaller mass of modified cardiac muscle cells located in the **interatrial septum,** just superior to the opening of the **coronary sinus.** The **AV bundle (of His)** arises from this node and lies within the **membranous portion of the interventricular septum.** It courses toward the apex of the heart, and at the upper portion of the muscular portion of this septum, it divides into **right and left bundle branches.** The bundle branches lie on their respective sides of the septum just beneath the endocardium. The bundles then divide to form a **subendocardial plexus of Purkinje fibers.** The right bundle is described as supplying the interventricular septum, the anterior papillary muscle (reached by the septomarginal or moderator band), and the wall of the right ventricle. The left bundle supplies the interventricular septum, anterior and posterior papillary muscles, and the wall of the left ventricle.

The SA node or pacemaker typically will depolarize at a rate of approximately 70 times per minute. This rate is referred to as a **sinus rhythm.** The SA node is innervated by fibers of the **sympathetic and parasympathetic divisions** of the autonomic nervous system. Stimulation of the SA node by sympathetic nerve impulses increases the rate of depolarization of the SA node, and stimulation by parasympathetic fibers decreases this rate.

Figure 13-1. Cardiac conduction system: 1 = sinoatrial node, 2 = anterior internodal pathway, 3 = middle internodal pathway (Wenckebach bundle), 4 = posterior internodal pathway, 5 = atrioventricular node, 6 = atrioventricular bundle of His, 7 = moderator band, 8 = right bundle branch, 9 = terminal conducting fibers of Purkinje, 10 = left bundle branch. (*Reproduced, with permission, from the University of Texas Health Science Center Houston Medical School.*)

Cardiac Valves

The outflow from the two atria and the two ventricles is guarded by the **AV and the semilunar valves,** respectively. The leaflets of these cardiac valves and the myocardial muscle fibers are attached to the **fibrous cardiac skeleton.** This structure consists of **four fibrous rings** to which the leaflets attach, the right and left fibrous trigone, and the membranous portion of the interventricular septum.

The right AV or tricuspid valve between the right atrium and right ventricle consists of anterior, posterior, and septal leaflets or cusps. Tendinous cords attach to the margins of adjacent valve cusps and prevent separation and inversion (prolapse) of the leaflets into the atrium during ventricular contraction. The proximal attachment of the tendinous cords is to conical projections of cardiac muscle called **papillary muscles;** there are three papillary muscles, named anterior, posterior, and septal, like the cusps. The **tendinous cords of the anterior papillary muscle** attach to the anterior and posterior cusps. Those of the posterior papillary muscle attach to the posterior and septal cusps, and the cords of the septal papillary muscle attach to the septal and anterior cusps.

The left AV or **bicuspid (mitral) valve** between the left atrium and ventricle consists of anterior and posterior cusps. The anterior and posterior papillary muscles, although larger due to the increased pressure demands, have their tendinous cords attached to adjacent cusps and function in a manner similarly described for the tricuspid valve.

The outflow from the right and left ventricles is guarded by the **pulmonary and aortic semilunar valves,** respectively. Both semilunar valves are similar in their structure, being circular in shape and consisting of three cup-like cusps, with the opening to these cups directed superiorly. The space formed is called the pulmonary or aortic sinus and is named for the cusp that creates it. As blood is ejected from the ventricles, the cusps lie close to the pulmonary or aortic wall. At the end of contraction, the elasticity of the vessel walls results in backflow of blood that fills the sinuses, resulting in apposition of the three cusps and closure of the valves. The cusps of the pulmonary semilunar valve are the anterior, right, and left cusps, and the aortic valve has right, left, and posterior cusps. The right and left coronary arteries arise from the aorta at the right and left aortic sinuses respectively.

COMPREHENSION QUESTIONS

[13.1] As a pathologist, you are examining the heart of a victim of fatal trauma and note a tear at the junction of the SVC and the right atrium. This tear would likely damage which of the following?

    A. SA node
    B. AV node
    C. AV bundle
    D. Right bundle branch
    E. Left bundle branch

[13.2] As a pathologist, you must examine the AV bundle histologically. In which of the following tissue samples will you find the AV bundle?

    A. Right atrium
    B. Left atrium
    C. Interatrial septum
    D. Membranous interventricular septum
    E. Muscular interventricular septum

[13.3] A 57-year-old man develops a myocardial infarction and is noted to
        have a heart rate of 40 beats/min. The cardiologist diagnoses an occlu-
        sion of the right coronary artery. Which of the following structures is
        most likely to be affected?

        A. AV node
        B. Bundle of His
        C. Purkinje fibers
        D. Mitral valve

Answers

[13.1] **A.** The SA node or pacemaker lies within the right atrial wall, where
        it is joined by the SVC.

[13.2] **D.** The AV bundle is located in the membranous portion of the inter-
        ventricular septum.

[13.3] **A.** An inferior wall myocardial infarction involving the right coronary
        artery may affect the AV node, leading to bradycardia.

ANATOMY PEARLS

❖ The cardiac conduction system is composed of specially modified
   cardiac muscle cells (not nervous tissue).
❖ The SA node is the pacemaker that spontaneously produces a sinus
   rhythm of 70 beats/min. It lies at the junction of the SVC and the
   right atrium.
❖ The AV node lies in the interatrial septum, and the AV bundle and
   the right and left bundle branches lie in the membranous and
   muscular portions of the interventricular septum, respectively.
❖ Stimulation of the SA node by sympathetic nerve impulses increases its
   rate of depolarization, whereas parasympathetic impulses decrease
   its rate.

REFERENCES

Moore KL, Dalley AF. Clinically Oriented Anatomy, 5th ed. Baltimore, MD:
    Lippincott Williams & Wilkins, 2006:147–50, 152–5, 162–3.
Netter FH. Atlas of Human Anatomy, 4th ed. Philadelphia, PA: Saunders, 2006:
    plates 222–3, 225.
Snell RS. Clinical Anatomy by Regions, 8th ed. Baltimore, MD: Lippincott
    Williams & Wilkins, 2008:105–13.

A 65-year-old woman underwent surgery to remove her uterus (total abdominal hysterectomy) due to uterine cancer 2 days previously. She was doing well until today, when she developed shortness of breath, and she describes a sharp pain in the right side of her chest at inspiration. On physical examination, her respiratory rate is 28 breaths/min and a heart rate of 110 beats/min. Auscultation of the lungs demonstrates no wheezing or crackles. She appears anxious.

◆ **What is the most likely diagnosis?**

◆ **What is the most likely location of the primary disease?**

ANSWERS TO CASE 14: PULMONARY EMBOLISM

Summary: Two days ago, a 65-year-old woman underwent a total abdominal hysterectomy due to endometrial cancer. She developed acute onset dyspnea with pleuritic chest pain. She has tachypnea and tachycardia and appears anxious. Rales (crackles) are not present by pulmonary examination.

◆ **Most likely diagnosis:** Pulmonary embolism

◆ **Most likely location of the primary disease:** Deep vein thrombosis (DVT) of the pelvis or lower limb

CLINICAL CORRELATION

This woman has multiple risk factors for DVT or blood clot formation within the large veins. These factors include the patient's age, likely minimal physical exercise, and bed rest after a major operative gynecological procedure for a cancerous lesion. Postoperative orthopedic patients are similarly at risk. Deep vein thrombi are typically asymptomatic but may cause lower limb swelling and pain. When pelvic or lower limb veins are involved, clot material can break free (embolize) and travel through the IVC to and through the right side of the heart, whence they are pumped to the lungs, where they will lodge in branches of the pulmonary arteries. These emboli effectively block blood flow beyond this point and prevent this unoxygenated blood from reaching the alveoli, where it is to be oxygenated. The size and number of emboli produced will determine the amount of lung tissue that will be infarcted due to lack of oxygen. The most common symptom of pulmonary embolism is dyspnea, and patients are often anxious, with tachycardia and pleuritic chest pain at inspiration. The next step would be an arterial blood-gas study to assess oxygen status. A chest radiograph and ventilation-perfusion scan are performed to directly determine whether an embolus is present. If present, intravenous anticoagulants such as heparin are beneficial. Large or untreated emboli can cause death. One particularly devastating type is called the saddle embolus. This type lodges in the pulmonary trunk at the bifurcation of the right and left pulmonary arteries, thus blocking blood flow to both lungs, leading to cardiovascular collapse and death.

APPROACH TO PULMONARY VASCULATURE

Objectives

1. Be able to describe the origin, branching pattern, and anatomical relations of the pulmonary arteries and the pulmonary veins.
2. Be able to describe the origin of the bronchial arteries, structures supplied, and sites of anastomosis with the pulmonary circulation.

Definitions

Total hysterectomy: Complete surgical removal of the uterus, that is, the body and the cervix. A subtotal hysterectomy consists of removal of the uterine corpus (body) but not of the cervix.

Pulmonary embolism: Obstruction or occlusion of pulmonary arteries by emboli typically arising from thrombi of veins in the lower limbs or the pelvis.

Infarction: Tissue necrosis due to the sudden decrease in the blood supply as the result of an embolus, thrombus, or external pressure.

Rales: "Crackles" heard when listening to the lung fields with a stethoscope, usually indicative of excess fluid in the lungs as with pneumonia or pulmonary edema.

DISCUSSION

The pulmonary trunk, which carries unoxygenated blood, arises from the **conus arteriosus** portion of the right ventricle. At the level of the sternal angle, the trunk divides into **right and left pulmonary arteries** (see Figure 14-1). The right pulmonary artery passes laterally, posterior to the ascending aorta and SVC, to reach the hilum of the right lung. The left pulmonary artery passes

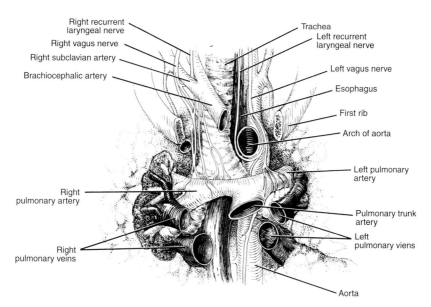

Figure 14-1. Superior mediastinum and relations of the pulmonary vessels. (*Reproduced, with permission, from Way LW, ed. Current Surgical Diagnosis and Treatment, 7th ed. East Norwalk, CT: Appleton & Lange, 1985.*)

anterior to the descending thoracic aorta to reach the hilum of the left lung. The pulmonary arteries are the most superior vessels in the hilum of each lung, and the branch to the superior lobe of each lung typically arises outside the lung hilum. Each artery courses through the lung tissue adjacent to bronchial and bronchiolar airway structures, where they branch out and are named for these airway structures. Thus each artery will divide into lobar and then segmental branches to the lung lobes and their **bronchopulmonary segments,** respectively. Further branching of **bronchioles** and the adjacent arteries occur down to the level of the **terminal bronchiole,** which supplies a lobule, the smallest anatomical unit of lung tissue.

As the small pulmonary artery branches reach the respiratory bronchioles, they form the extensive capillary network around and between the alveoli. **The thin capillary endothelium, basal lamina, and type I pneumocytes form the blood-gas barrier through which gaseous exchange occurs.**

Oxygenated blood drains from the capillary bed to pulmonary veins within the thin connective tissue septae between lobules. In this location, they receive blood from adjacent lobules. As the pulmonary veins unite to form increasingly larger veins, they remain separated from the pulmonary artery and airway structures, being found at the periphery of lung tissue subdivisions such as the bronchopulmonary segments and lobes. These larger veins will drain adjacent segments or lobes. Eventually, two pulmonary veins exit the hilum of each lung anteriorly and inferiorly to the entering pulmonary arteries. Thus **four pulmonary veins** drain oxygenated blood into the left atrium.

The **bronchi, bronchioles,** and related structures, the connective tissue stroma and the visceral pleura, receive their blood supply from bronchial arteries. These are typically branches of the **thoracic aorta** but may arise from intercostal arteries. Anastomoses between the pulmonary and bronchial arteries occur within the bronchial walls and the visceral pleura. Bronchial veins from the right and left lungs typically drain to the azygous and accessory hemiazygous veins, respectively, but carry only small amounts of blood. The pulmonary vein carries most of the blood supplied by the bronchial arteries.

COMPREHENSION QUESTIONS

[14.1] As a surgeon exploring the thorax, you will be able to identify the right pulmonary artery in which of the following locations?

    A. Anterior to the ascending aorta and the SVC
    B. Anterior to the ascending aorta and posterior to the SVC
    C. Posterior to the descending aorta and the SVC
    D. Posterior to the ascending aorta and the SVC
    E. Posterior to the ascending aorta and anterior to the SVC

[14.2] As a radiologist examining a contrast study of the pulmonary vessels, you will note how many pulmonary veins entering the left atrium?

    A. Two
    B. Three
    C. Four
    D. Five
    E. Six

[14.3] A 44-year-old woman who has a DVT of the lower extremity suddenly gasps and collapses. She is found to be hypotensive. Resuscitative measures are attempted without success. Which of the following is the most likely diagnosis?

    A. Myocardial infarction
    B. Saddle embolus
    C. Right peripheral pulmonary embolus
    D. Embolic stroke

Answers

[14.1] **D.** The right pulmonary passes posteriorly to the ascending aorta and the SVC.

[14.2] **C.** Four pulmonary veins that carry oxygenated blood drain into the left atrium.

[14.3] **B.** The patient likely developed a saddle embolus that occluded blood flow to both pulmonary arteries and, in effect, stopped the circulatory system.

> ## ANATOMY PEARLS
>
> Pulmonary arteries carry unoxygenated blood, accompany airway structures, and follow their branching patterns; pulmonary veins, which carry oxygenated blood, course separately from the arteries and airways at the periphery of lung tissue subdivisions.
> The blood-gas barrier is composed of the capillary endothelium, basal lamina, and type I pneumocytes.
> Bronchial arteries typically arise from the thoracic aorta and supply the airway structures and stromal tissue.

REFERENCES

Moore KL, Dalley AF. Clinically Oriented Anatomy, 5th ed. Baltimore, MD: Lippincott Williams & Wilkins, 2006:129–31.

Netter FH. Atlas of Human Anatomy, 4th ed. Philadelphia, PA: Saunders, 2006: plates 205–7.

Snell RS. Clinical Anatomy by Regions, 8th ed. Baltimore, MD: Lippincott Williams & Wilkins, 2008:126.

A 54-year-old man who had smoked two packs of cigarettes per day for 20 years complains of the acute onset of shortness of breath, and severe chest pain with respiratory movement. On physical examination, he has a barrel chest consistent with chronic obstructive pulmonary disease. There are decreased breath sounds on the right side. When the physician taps on the right chest (percussion), there is a hyperresonant (unusually hollow) sound.

◆ **What is the most likely diagnosis?**

◆ **What is the anatomical disorder?**

ANSWERS TO CASE 15: PNEUMOTHORAX

Summary: A 54-year-old smoker complains of acute onset of shortness of breath and severe chest pain with breathing. He has physical findings for chronic obstructive pulmonary disease with a barrel chest. There are decreased breath sounds and hyperresonance to percussion on the right side.

◆ **Most likely diagnosis:** Pneumothorax

◆ **Anatomical disorder:** Entry of air into the pleural space, resulting in lung collapse

CLINICAL CORRELATION

Air is drawn into the lungs through the trachea and bronchi by the increasing negative thoracic pressure produced by the downward movement of the diaphragm. If air enters the pleural space through the thoracic wall or the surface of the lung itself, the negative pressure of the pleural space equilibrates with atmospheric pressure, and air movement ceases. The defect that allowed air to enter the pleural space acts like a valve by preventing the air from exiting the space. Pressure increases above that of atmospheric pressure, and a tension pneumothorax results, which is characterized by lung collapse, with displacement toward the mediastinum. If severe enough, the mediastinum and its contents may be displaced toward the intact lung and produce partial compression of this lung. The most serious consequence of these anatomical shifts is decreased venous return to the heart. This patient who has chronic obstructive pulmonary disease is at risk for spontaneous pneumothorax by the rupture of an emphysematous bleb on the surface of the lung. Spontaneous pneumothorax may also occur from lung surface blebs in young men. The typical clinical presentation of pneumothorax is chest pain with dyspnea, decreased breath sounds, and hyperresonance on the affected side. The diagnosis is confirmed by chest radiograph. Treatment is directed toward removal of the air from the pleural space with a needle in emergent situations or by a chest tube placed in the pleural space and directed to an underwater seal.

APPROACH TO THE PLEURAL CAVITIES

Objectives

1. Be able to describe the contents of the pulmonary cavities: lungs and the pleural divisions.
2. Be able to describe the superior and inferior limits of the pleural cavity and the lower limits of each lung.
3. Be able to describe the functional importance of the pleural cavity and fluid and the pressure within the cavity.

Definitions

Chronic obstructive pulmonary disease: General term applied to permanent or temporary diseases that cause narrowing of the bronchi so as to obstruct forced expiratory flow and includes bronchitis, emphysema, asthma, among others.

Emphysema: A lung condition in which the air spaces distal to the terminal bronchioles are larger than normal.

Pneumothorax: Air or gas within the pleural cavity.

Chest tube: Tube inserted through the thoracic wall into the pleural cavity for the purpose of draining air or fluid from that cavity.

DISCUSSION

The **skeletal components of the thoracic wall** are the thoracic vertebra, the attached **12 pairs of ribs and the sternum.** The interval between the ribs is closed by three layers of muscles, the **external, internal, and innermost intercostal muscles.** The transverse thoracic and subcostal muscles are discontinuous thoracic wall muscles found anteriorly and posteriorly, respectively. Externally, several muscles associated with the upper limb or accessory respiratory muscles attach to the thoracic wall. These include the pectoralis major and minor, serratus anterior and posterior, scalene, and levator costarum muscles. Internally, the thoracic cavity is divided into two pulmonary cavities separated by the central **mediastinum.** The thoracic cavity is closed inferiorly by the diaphragm.

Each of the two laterally placed pulmonary cavities contains a lung covered with visceral pleura, and each is lined with parietal pleura. The two pleura are continuous with each other at the root of the lung, where neurovascular and airway structures enter and exit the lung. The pleura is a serous membrane composed of mesothelium and a small amount of connective tissue, and it produces the lubricating pleural fluid. The parietal pleura is divided for descriptive purposes into four parts based on the structure to which it is attached. The costal, diaphragmatic, mediastinal, and cervical portions are attached, respectively, to the inner aspect of the thoracic wall, the superior surface of the diaphragm, the lateral aspect of the mediastinum, especially the pericardial sac, and the root of the neck superior to the superior thoracic aperture.

Relative constant pleural lines of reflection are created as one portion of parietal pleura changes direction to attach to another structure (Figure 15-1). The **sternal reflection line** is created as the mediastinal pleura change direction (is reflected) onto the inner thoracic wall and become the costal pleura. In the right pulmonary cavity, this line of reflection is close to the midline from the sternal angle to the xiphoid process. On the left side, the line of reflection courses from the sternal angle to the level of the fourth rib, and then arches to the left to the sixth rib in the midclavicular line, thus creating the cardiac notch. Due to the curvature of the mediastinal surface in this region, a shallow

Figure 15-1. The lungs (bounded by solid line) and pleura (denoted by the heavy dotted line). (*Reproduced, with permission, from the University of Texas Health Science Center Houston Medical School.*)

costomediastinal recess of the pleural cavity is created. Inferiorly as the **costal pleura** are reflected onto the surface of the diaphragm, the costal reflection line is created. The surface landmarks for this reflection line on the right and left sides are the 8th rib at the midclavicular line (MCL), the 10th rib at the midaxillary line (MAL), and the 12th rib at the vertebral border. These landmarks also mark the inferior limits of the pleural cavity. The curved shape of the diaphragmatic pleura on the dome of the diaphragm and the vertical costal pleura form a wedge-shaped pleural cavity recess called the **costodiaphragmatic recess,** in which abnormal pleural cavity fluids such as blood or pus will accumulate. The lowest level of each lung at the end of expiration is the 6th rib at the MCL, the 8th rib at the MAL, and the 10th rib at the vertebral border. The cervical pleura and thus the pleural cavity extend into the root of the neck, 2 to 3 cm superior to the medial end of the clavicle.

The **pleural cavity between the visceral and parietal layers of pleura** is a potential space in which there is a small amount of lubricating pleural fluid.

This fluid wets the surface of the lungs, resulting in adherence of the lung's visceral pleura to the costal and diaphragmatic parietal pleura by surface tension forces. As the diaphragm descends and the thoracic wall expands with inspiration, the adherent lungs also expand. The pleural cavities are completely closed spaces and are at 756 mm Hg of pressure, or at –4 mm Hg with respect to atmospheric pressure (760 mm Hg). If the visceral pleura covering the lung is ruptured or the costal parietal pleura is disrupted by trauma, air will enter the pleural cavity, causing a **pneumothorax** and at least equalizing pleural pressure with atmospheric pressure. This will produce at least a partial lung collapse and interfere with ventilation and gaseous exchange.

COMPREHENSION QUESTIONS

[15.1] You must remove fluid from the pleural cavity of your patient (thoracentesis). You decide to insert the aspiration needle over the top of a rib, into an intercostal space inferior to the lower border of the lung in the MAL at the end of a normal expiration. Which of the following is the highest level at which this procedure might safely be done without injuring the lung?

   A. Fourth intercostal space
   B. Fifth intercostal space
   C. Sixth intercostal space
   D. Seventh intercostal space
   E. Eighth intercostal space

[15.2] While performing this thoracentesis procedure, the lowest level of the pleural cavity will lie at the level of which rib at the end of expiration in the MAL?

   A. Seventh
   B. Eighth
   C. Ninth
   D. Tenth
   E. Eleventh

[15.3] While performing this procedure, the lower border of the lung will lie at the level of which rib in the MCL?

   A. Fifth
   B. Sixth
   C. Seventh
   D. Eighth
   E. Ninth

Answers

[15.1]   **E.** The lower border of the lung will lie at the level of the eighth rib in the MAL, so the needle can be safely inserted into the eighth intercostal space.

[15.2]   **D.** The lowest level of the pleural cavity in the MAL lies at the level of the 10th rib.

[15.3]   **B.** The lower border of the lung at the MCL at the level of the sixth rib.

ANATOMY PEARLS

❖ Visceral and parietal pleura are continuous with each other at the root of the lung.

❖ The inferior extent of the pleural cavity is the 6th rib at the MCL line, 8th rib at the MAL, and 10th rib at the vertebral border.

❖ The inferior border of each lung at the end of expiration is the 8th rib at the midclavicular line, 10th rib at the MAL, and 12th rib at the vertebral border.

❖ The pleural cavity is at −4 mm Hg with respect to atmospheric pressure.

REFERENCES

Moore KL, Dalley AF. Clinically Oriented Anatomy, 5th ed. Baltimore, MD: Lippincott Williams & Wilkins, 2006:112–23.

Netter FH. Atlas of Human Anatomy, 4th ed. Philadelphia, PA: Saunders, 2006: plates 196–8.

Snell RS. Clinical Anatomy by Regions, 8th ed. Baltimore, MD: Lippincott Williams & Wilkins, 2008:80–5, 89–96.

A 59-year-old man complains of tight chest pressure and shortness of breath after lifting several boxes in his garage approximately 2 hours ago. He says he believes his heart is skipping beats. His medical history is significant for hypertension and cigarette smoking. On examination, his heart rate is 55 beats/min and regular, and his lungs are clear to auscultation. An electrocardiogram shows bradycardia with an increased PR interval and ST-segment elevation in multiple leads including the anterior leads, V1 and V2.

◆ **What is the most likely diagnosis?**

◆ **What anatomical structures are most likely affected?**

ANSWERS TO CASE 16: CORONARY ARTERY DISEASE

Summary: A 59-year-old hypertensive male smoker has a 2-hour history of tight chest pressure, shortness of breath, and palpitations after exertion. His heart rate is 55 beats/min and regular. The electrocardiogram (ECG) shows bradycardia, first-degree heart block, and ST-segment elevation in leads V1 and V2.

◆ **Most likely diagnosis:** Myocardial infarction

◆ **Anatomical structures likely affected:** Right coronary artery and left anterior descending artery

CLINICAL CORRELATION

This patient's 2-hour history of worsening chest pain, dyspnea, and palpitations after physical exertion is classic for a myocardial infarction. The pain of angina due to the myocardial ischemia is typically deep, visceral, and squeezing in nature, like an "elephant stepping on the chest." It frequently radiates to the neck or left arm. This patient's risk factors include hypertension and tobacco use. The ECG (ST-segment elevation) is highly suspicious for myocardial infarction. Leads V1 and V2 are used to evaluate the anterior portion of the heart which is supplied by the left anterior descending artery. Bradycardia and first-degree heart block (increased PR interval) indicate right coronary artery disease.

APPROACH TO CORONARY ARTERY CIRCULATION

Objectives

1. Be able to describe the course and areas of the heart supplied by the right and left coronary arteries, respectively.
2. Be able to describe the venous drainage of the heart.
3. Be able to describe the arterial supply and venous drainage of the pericardial sac.

Definitions

Angina: Chest pain classically described as pressure or "squeezing" indicative of coronary artery insufficiency and cardiac ischemia.
Ischemia: Inadequate blood supply and oxygen delivery to tissue.
Palpitations: Pulsations of the heart perceptible by a patient that are usually irregular and increased in force.
Bradycardia: Heart rate no faster than 60 beats/min.

DISCUSSION

The **heart** receives its **arterial blood supply** from the **first branches of the ascending aorta,** the **right and left coronary arteries.** The right and left artery arise from the aorta at the aortic sinuses, the pockets formed by the right and left cusps of the aortic valve, respectively. Each artery will supply portions of the atria and ventricles.

The **right coronary artery (RCA)** arises at the right aortic sinus and courses in the coronary (AV) groove between the right atrium and ventricle. At the level of the right auricular appendage, it gives off the SA nodal branch, which ascends to the junction of the SVC with the right atrium, where the SA node is located. As it reaches the inferior margin of the heart in the coronary groove, it will usually give off a right marginal branch that supplies the right ventricle along the inferior border. The RCA then curves around the inferior margin of the heart in the coronary groove onto the inferior and posterior surfaces of the heart, passing somewhat to the left toward the junction with the posterior interventricular groove, also called the crux of the heart. At the crux, the AV nodal branch passes deep into the interatrial septum to supply the AV node. The RCA divides into a larger posterior interventricular artery, which descends in the groove or sulcus of the same name. It passes toward but typically does not reach the apex of the heart. It supplies the right and left ventricles and posterior portions of the interventricular septum. A small branch continues to the left side of the heart to supply portions of the left atrium and ventricle and will anastomose with the circumflex branch of the left coronary artery (LCA; Figures 16-1 and 16-2).

Figure 16-1. Anterior view of the heart: 1 = aortic arch, 2 = superior vena cava, 3 = pulmonary trunk, 4 = right auricle, 5 = right atrium, 6 = coronary sulcus and vessels, 7 = epicardial fat, 8 = inferior vena cava, 9 = right ventricle, 10 = ligamentum arteriosum, 11 = left auricle, 12 = left ventricle, 13 = anterior interventricular sulcus and vessels. (*Reproduced, with permission, from the University of Texas Health Science Center Houston Medical School.*)

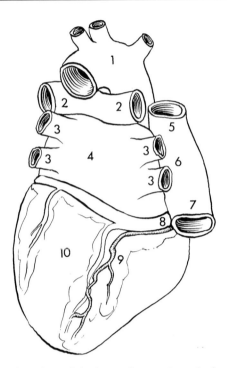

Figure 16-2. Posterior view of the heart: 1 = aortic arch, 2 = pulmonary arteries, 3 = pulmonary veins, 4 = left atrium, 5 = superior vena cava, 6 = right atrium,
7 = inferior vena cava, 8 = coronary sinus, 9 = posterior interventricular sulcus
and vessels, 10 = left ventricle. (*Reproduced, with permission, from the
University of Texas Health Science Center Houston Medical School.*)

The **LCA** arises from the left aortic sinus and quickly bifurcates into an
anterior interventricular and circumflex arteries. The anterior interventricular
or left anterior descending (LAD) artery descends toward the apex of the heart
in the anterior interventricular groove, where it curves around the apex onto the
diaphragmatic surface of the heart to anastomose with the posterior (descending)
interventricular branch of the RCA. The anterior interventricular artery supplies
the anterior portion of the right and left ventricles and anterior two-thirds of the
interventricular septum and therefore is the chief blood supply to the AV and
the right and left bundles of the heart's conducting system. The other smaller
branch of the LCA is the **circumflex branch,** which travels in the coronary
groove toward the left margin of the heart, at which point it typically gives off
a left marginal branch that supplies the left heart border portion of the left ventricle. The circumflex artery curves around the left heart border to anastomose
with the RCA at the posterior aspects of the left atrium and ventricle. The pattern of arterial blood supply at this point is often described as a balanced blood

supply because the RCA and LCA supply approximately equal amounts to the heart. In approximately 15 percent of the population, the LCA will supply a larger proportion than the RCA.

The majority of **venous blood will enter the right atrium** through the coronary sinus, which lies in the coronary groove on the posterior surface of the heart. Its internal opening is adjacent to the opening of the IVC. Great, middle, and small cardiac veins and several smaller named veins drain into the coronary sinus. A variable number of small anterior cardiac veins drain directly into the right atrium. The smallest cardiac veins drain small amounts of blood from the myocardial capillary plexus directly into the atria and ventricles.

The heart's **pericardial sac** receives its arterial blood supply primarily from the **pericardiacophrenic artery** (a branch of the internal thoracic artery) that accompanies the phrenic nerve. Small amounts of arterial blood are also provided by branches of the musculophrenic, superior phrenic, bronchial, and esophageal arteries. Pericardiacophrenic veins drain blood to the internal thoracic or brachiocephalic veins.

COMPREHENSION QUESTIONS

[16.1] As a cardiologist, you are concerned about blockage of the artery to the SA node in a patient. This artery typically arises from which of the following?

A. RCA
B. Right marginal artery
C. Posterior interventricular artery
D. Anterior interventricular artery
E. Circumflex artery

[16.2] In a balanced coronary artery pattern, the blood supply to the majority of the interventricular septum is derived from which of the following?

A. RCA
B. AV artery
C. Posterior interventricular artery
D. Anterior interventricular artery
E. Circumflex artery

[16.3] As a cardiologist, you are concerned about blockage of the artery to the AV node in a patient. This artery typically arises from which of the following?

A. RCA
B. Right marginal artery
C. Posterior interventricular artery
D. Anterior interventricular artery
E. Circumflex artery

Answers

[16.1]   **A.** The SA node is typically supplied by the RCA.

[16.2]   **D.** Usually, the anterior two-thirds of the interventricular septum is supplied by the AV artery, and the right and left bundle branches of the conduction system are generally supplied by the anterior interventricular artery.

[16.3]   **A.** The AV node is also supplied by the RCA.

ANATOMY PEARLS

 In a balanced coronary circulation as described above, the conduction system nodes of the heart (SA and AV nodes) are typically supplied by the RCA.

 In a balanced coronary circulation, the anastomoses between branches of the RCA and LCA occur at the posterior coronary and posterior interventricular grooves.

 Most cardiac veins drain into the coronary sinus, which opens into the right atrium adjacent to the opening of the IVC.

REFERENCES

Moore KL, Dalley AF. Clinically Oriented Anatomy, 5th ed. Baltimore, MD: Lippincott Williams & Wilkins, 2006:156–62.

Netter FH. Atlas of Human Anatomy, 4th ed. Philadelphia, PA: Saunders, 2006: plates 216–9.

Snell RS. Clinical Anatomy by Regions, 8th ed. Baltimore, MD: Lippincott Williams & Wilkins, 2008:113–6.

A 31-year-old woman with one healthy child presents with a 2-year history of an inability to conceive. She states that her menstrual periods began at age 12 and occur at regular 28-day intervals. A biphasic basal body temperature chart is recorded. She denies having any sexually transmitted disease, and a hysterosalpingogram shows patent uterine tubes and a normal uterine cavity. Her husband is 34 years old and his semen analysis is normal. In the presence of several normal test results for infertility, a laparoscopic examination of the pelvic cavity is scheduled. The physician performing the procedure carefully places the trocar lateral to the rectus abdominis muscle and its sheath to avoid injury to a major artery.

◆ **What artery is being avoided?**

◆ **What is the anatomical location of this structure?**

ANSWERS TO CASE 17: INFERIOR EPIGASTRIC ARTERY

Summary: An infertile couple is being evaluated, and several tests for infertility have shown normal results. A laparoscopic examination of the pelvic cavity is performed to rule out the presence of endometriosis. The trocar is specifically placed lateral to the rectus abdominis muscle and its sheath to avoid a major artery.

◆ **Artery that is avoided:** Inferior epigastric artery

◆ **Anatomical location of this artery:** Posterior to the rectus abdominis within the rectus sheath

CLINICAL CORRELATION

The presence of several normal test results indicates a need to rule out endometriosis in this infertile couple. Endometriosis is defined as ectopic endometrial tissue outside the uterus, typically adherent to the pelvic peritoneum. This tissue responds to a woman's hormonal cycles in the same way that the lining of the uterus responds. Although the mechanism is not fully understood, endometriosis may cause infertility by inhibiting ovulation, producing adhesions, or interfering with fertilization. Laparoscopic examination of the pelvic cavity is indicated and, if possible at this time, ablation of the endometrial tissue.

APPROACH TO ANTERIOR ABDOMINAL WALL

Objectives

1. Be able to describe the arterial blood supply of the anterior abdominal wall.
2. Be able to describe the relation of these vessels to the musculature of the anterior abdominal wall, including the rectus sheath.

Definitions

Biphasic basal body temperature chart: Elevation of the oral temperature during the second half of the menstrual cycle indicating that the patient has ovulated.

Hysterosalpingogram: Radiologic study in which radiopaque dye is injected into the uterine lumen through a transcervical catheter to evaluate the uterine cavity or the patency of the uterine tubes.

Laparoscopy: Surgical technique to visualize the peritoneal cavity through a rigid telescopic instrument called a laparoscope.

Endometriosis: Condition in which the lining tissue of the uterus, the endometrium, is far outside the uterus, typically in the pelvic cavity or on the abdominal wall.

DISCUSSION

The **anterior abdominal** wall is composed of three paired flat muscles that, in general, arise from bony structures posteriorly and whose fibrous aponeuroses form the rectus sheath and meet to form the **linea alba.** These muscles are from superficial to deep: the **external abdominal oblique, internal abdominal oblique, and transversus abdominis (Figure 17-1).** These muscles are supplied by segmental branches of the thoracic and abdominal aorta: the 10th, 11th, and 12th (subcostal) intercostal arteries and the 1st or 2nd lumbar arteries. These **arteries,** their companion **veins, and the nerves** supplying the muscles are all found **in the interval between the internal abdominal oblique and the transversus abdominis muscles,** known as the **neurovascular plane. Superficial and deep circumflex iliac arteries** arise from the **femoral and external iliac arteries,** respectively, course parallel to the inguinal ligament, and supply the inferior abdominal wall in the inguinal region. The superficial epigastric arteries lie in the superficial fascia between the umbilicus and the pubic bone. The internal thoracic arteries divide into two terminal branches: the superior epigastric and musculophrenic arteries (Figure 17-2).

External oblique
Anterior rectus sheath
Transversus abdominis
Position of curvilinear line of Douglas (arcuate line)
Internal oblique
Transversalis fascia

Tendinous intersection
Rectus abdominis
Pyramidalis

Figure 17-1. Muscles of the anterior abdominal wall. (*Reproduced, with permission, from Lindner HH. Clinical Anatomy. East Norwalk, CT:Appleton & Lange, 1989:291.*)

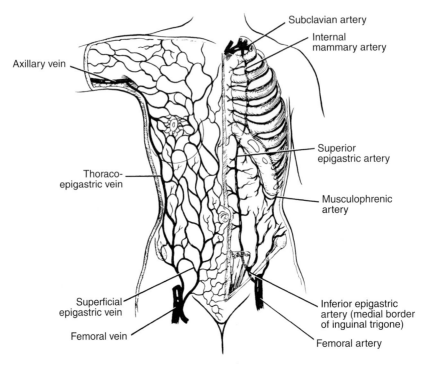

Figure 17-2. Arteries of the anterior abdominal wall. (*Reproduced, with permission, from Lindner HH. Clinical Anatomy. East Norwalk, CT:Appleton & Lange, 1989:299.*)

The anterior central region of the abdominal wall is formed by the paired **rectus abdominis** muscles, which attach to the pubic bone inferiorly and the rib cartilages superiorly, and lie just lateral to the linea alba. Each muscle is subdivided into short belly segments by typically three or more tendinous inscriptions. Each muscle is contained in a fibrous compartment, the **rectus sheath,** that is formed by the aponeuroses of the three flat abdominal muscles. Enclosing the superior three-fourths of each rectus muscle are anterior and posterior layers to the sheath. In this region, the aponeurosis of the internal abdominal muscle divides, and portions will pass anteriorly and posteriorly to the rectus muscle. It follows that the aponeuroses of the external oblique muscle and the transversus abdominis muscles **must pass anteriorly and posteriorly to the rectus, respectively.** At about the midpoint between the umbilicus and the pubic bone, the aponeuroses of all three flat abdominal muscles pass anterior to the rectus sheath; therefore, the inferior one-fourth of the rectus muscle has only an anterior rectus sheath. The inferior margin of the posterior rectus sheath can be identified in this region of transition as the **arcuate line.** The rectus sheath also contains the pyramidalis muscles, superior and inferior epigastric vessels, and terminations of the intercostal nerves that innervate the abdominal muscle. The superior one-fourth of the rectus muscle is supplied by the medial terminal branch of the **internal thoracic artery, the superior epigastric artery.** The **inferior epigastric artery** arises from the **external iliac artery** just before its exit from the abdomen to become the femoral artery. Each artery courses medially, external to the peritoneum, along the posterior surface of the rectus muscles. The superior and inferior epigastric arteries anastomose about half-way between the umbilicus and the xiphoid process.

COMPREHENSION QUESTIONS

[17.1] A surgeon entering the abdominal cavity through the abdominal wall will take care to avoid injury to the vessels and nerves within the wall. The main portion of these vessels and nerves will be found immediately deep to which of the following?

   A. Skin
   B. Superficial fascia
   C. External abdominal oblique muscle
   D. Internal abdominal oblique muscle
   E. Transversus abdominis muscle

[17.2] As a surgeon performing an appendectomy, you encounter an artery and vein in the superficial fascia of the lower abdominal wall. These vessels are most likely which of the following?

   A. Superficial epigastric artery and vein
   B. Superficial circumflex iliac artery and vein
   C. Intercostal artery and vein
   D. Inferior epigastric artery and vein
   E. Superior epigastric artery and vein

[17.3] During surgery, you must incise the anterior rectus sheath between the xiphoid process and the umbilicus. In this region, the sheath is derived from the aponeurosis of which of the following?

   A. External abdominal oblique only
   B. Internal abdominal oblique only
   C. External and internal abdominal oblique
   D. Internal oblique and transversus abdominis
   E. Transversus abdominis only

[17.4] During a laparoscopic procedure, you observe the inferior epigastric vessels ascending on the posterior surface of the rectus abdominis muscle. They suddenly disappear from view by passing superior to which of the following?

   A. Falx inguinalis
   B. Linea semilunaris
   C. Falciform ligament
   D. Arcuate line
   E. Transversalis fascia

Answers

[17.1] **D.** The main course of the intercostal vessels and nerves is deep to the internal abdominal oblique muscle in the neurovascular plane.

[17.2] **A.** The superficial epigastric vessels lie within the superficial fascia.

[17.3] **C.** The superior three-fourths of the anterior rectus sheath is derived from the aponeuroses of the external and internal abdominal oblique muscles.

[17.4] **D.** As the inferior epigastric vessels ascend on the posterior surface of the rectus abdominis muscle, they will pass superiorly to the arcuate line, anteriorly to the posterior rectus sheath.

ANATOMY PEARLS

 The neurovascular plane of the anterolateral abdominal wall lies deep to the internal abdominal oblique muscle.

 Along the superior three-fourths of the rectus muscles, the internal oblique aponeurosis splits to contribute to the anterior and posterior rectus sheath layers.

 The inferior epigastric artery arises from the external iliac artery, lies on the posterior surface of the rectus muscle, and is its main blood supply.

REFERENCES

Moore KL, Dalley AF. Clinically Oriented Anatomy, 5th ed. Baltimore, MD: Lippincott Williams & Wilkins, 2006:196–213.

Netter FH. Atlas of Human Anatomy, 4th ed. Philadelphia, PA: Saunders, 2006: plates 251, 255.

Snell, RS. Clinical Anatomy by Regions, 8th ed. Baltimore, MD: Lippincott Williams & Wilkins, 2008:146–52, 159–62.

A 44-year-old man complains of discomfort in his right upper thigh over the past 6 months. He works in the garden department of a home improvement center. On examination, there is tenderness at the right inguinal area. When the patient performs a Valsalva maneuver (bearing down to increase intra-abdominal pressure), a bulge appears superior to the inguinal crease near the pubic bone.

◆ **What is the most likely diagnosis?**

◆ **What is the anatomical defect associated with this condition?**

ANSWERS TO CASE 18: INGUINAL HERNIA

Summary: A 44-year-old man who works in the garden department of a home improvement center has a 6-month history of right groin pain. There is inguinal tenderness and a bulge with the performance of a Valsalva maneuver.

◆ **Most likely diagnosis:** Inguinal hernia

◆ **Associated anatomical defect:** Protrusion of an abdominal organ into the inguinal canal

CLINICAL CORRELATION

A hernia is defined as an abnormal protrusion of a structure through tissues that normally contain it. Inguinal hernias are the most common type of hernia, occurring in men and women, but occur much more frequently in men. This patient's age and his occupation, which requires frequent lifting activity, suggest a direct or acquired inguinal hernia. Loss of tone in the musculature in the inguinal region predisposes to progressive stretching of the parietal peritoneum into the posterior inguinal canal with repeated increased intra-abdominal pressure associated with the lifting activity. If the patient were a young man or child, an indirect or congenital inguinal hernia would be a more likely diagnosis. With an indirect hernia, the parietal peritoneum at the deep inguinal ring exists as a finger-like protrusion into the inguinal canal. This is the result of faulty closure of the embryonic outpouching of peritoneum into the scrotum, called the process vaginalis. Indirect inguinal hernias enter the deep inguinal ring, stretch peritoneal tissue with repeated increases in intra-abdominal pressure, traverse the length of the inguinal canal, and enter the scrotum. Surgical repair of the tissue defect is indicated to prevent incarceration, infarction, and necrosis of the herniated tissue, typically a loop of small intestine.

APPROACH TO THE INGUINAL REGION

Objectives

1. Be able to describe the anatomy of the inguinal region.
2. Be able to discern the anatomical basis for an indirect versus a direct inguinal hernial classification.

Definitions

Valsalva maneuver: Increase intra-abdominal pressure by attempting to exhale with a closed glottis.

DISCUSSION

The **inguinal region** is the junction between the **lower anterior abdominal** and the **upper anterior thigh.** It is the site at which several structures enter and exit the abdomen and therefore is an area of potential weakness in males and females. The **inguinal (Poupart) ligament** is an important anatomical structure and key landmark for this region. It is the thickened, rolled underedge of the inferior portion of the **external abdominal oblique aponeurosis.** It extends from the **anterior superior iliac spine** to the **pubic tubercle** and fuses inferiorly with the **fascia lata (deep fascia)** of the anterior thigh. At the pubic tubercle, the inguinal ligament continues posterolaterally on the **superior pubic ramus** (pectin of the pubic bone) as the **pectineal (Cooper) ligament.** At the point where these two ligaments are continuous and change directions, a ligamentous reflection fills the interval, forming the **lacunar (Gimbernat) ligament.**

The lacunar ligament forms a rigid medial margin for the femoral ring, leading to the femoral canal, the site for femoral hernias (Figure 18-1).

Although the external abdominal oblique muscle and aponeurosis comprise an essentially complete musculotendinous structure (except the superficial inguinal ring), the **internal abdominal oblique** and **transversus abdominis muscles** are deficient because they originate from the iliopsoas fascia and arch medially to their **tendinous (falx inguinalis) insertions on the pubic tubercle** (Figure 18-2).

Structures enter and exit the abdomen superior to the inguinal ligament through an oblique passage known as the **inguinal canal.** The canal is frequently described as a tunnel, with openings, walls, floor, and so on. These boundary features are listed in Table 18-1.

Inferior epigastric artery and vein

Rectus abdominis muscle

Hesselbach's area

Femoral ring

Lacunar ligament
Pectineal line of os pubis

Abberant obturator artery

Inguinal ligament

Deep inguinal ring

Femoral nerve
Iliopsoas muscle
External iliac artery

External iliac vein

Pectineal ligament

Ductus deferens

Figure 18-1. Inner surface of Hesselbach triangle. (*Reproduced, with permission, from Lindner HH. Clinical Anatomy. East Norwalk, CT:Appleton & Lange, 1989:288.*)

Figure 18-2. The ilioinguinal region. (*Reproduced, with permission, from Lindner HH. Clinical Anatomy. East Norwalk, CT: Appleton & Lange, 1989:291.*)

Two points in Table 18-1 are of anatomical and clinical significance. First, due to the arching of the internal oblique and transversus abdominis muscles, the **posterior wall of the canal is deficient and weak,** being formed only by the **transversalis fascia** and parietal peritoneum. However, with increased intra-abdominal pressure (as in lifting, bowel movement, etc.), these muscles contract and descend in a shutter-like fashion, thus reinforcing the posterior wall. Second, the outpouching of the transversalis fascia to form the **deep inguinal ring occurs immediately laterally to the inferior epigastric vessels** (see Case 17 for a discussion of their course). In addition, at the medial

Table 18-1

BOUNDARIES OF THE INGUINAL CANAL

ANTERIOR WALL	POSTERIOR WALL	FLOOR	ROOF	EXTERNAL OPENING	INTERNAL OPENING
Aponeurosis of external abdominal oblique muscle	Transversalis fascia and parietal peritoneum	Inguinal ligament and lacunar ligament medially	Arching fibers of internal oblique and transversus abdominis muscle	Superficial inguinal ring: triangular opening in external oblique aponeurosis	Site of outpouching of transversalis fascia: covered with parietal peritoneum

portion of the inguinal ligament on the interior of the abdominal wall, a clinically important **inguinal (Hesselbach) triangle** is formed by some of these structures. This triangle is formed by the **inguinal ligament, inferior epigastric vessels, and the lateral margin of the rectus abdominis muscle** and corresponds to the area where the posterior wall of the canal is deficient due to the arching of the abdominal wall muscles described above.

In **females,** the **inguinal canal is traversed by the round ligament of the uterus;** in **males, the spermatic cord (ductus deferens and associated vessels and nerves)** passes through the canal. The **ilioinguinal nerve** is found in the canal in both sexes.

The inguinal region and canal comprise the site for inguinal hernias. Although hernias occur in both sexes, they are far more common in males. There are two types of inguinal hernias, indirect and direct. **Indirect or congenital inguinal hernias tend to occur in young males**. During embryonic descent of the testes, an outpouching of **parietal peritoneum, the tunica vaginalis,** pushes through the lower abdominal wall, encountering first the transversalis fascia (thus forming the deep inguinal ring), slipping inferior to the transverses abdominis muscle, but catching the lower margin of the internal abdominal oblique muscle, and then pushing through the external abdominal oblique muscle **(forming the superficial inguinal ring).** The testes descend into the scrotum along the path created by the tunica vaginalis (and the gubernaculum). In normal development, this outpouching fuses and closes. If it does not fuse and close, a predisposing complete or partial path for the abnormal migration of an abdominal organ (usually small intestine) is established. The loop of small intestine would pass through the deep inguinal ring, inguinal canal, and possibly through the superficial ring into the scrotum. By definition, **indirect inguinal hernias** leave the abdominal cavity **lateral** to the **inferior epigastric vessels** (through the deep inguinal ring).

Direct inguinal hernias are also called acquired inguinal hernias because they are seen in older males and are related to strenuous activity that increases intra-abdominal pressure. It is believed that with aging there is loss of tone in the abdominal musculature and the shutter-like actions described above for the internal abdominal oblique and transverses abdominis are diminished or lost. This predisposes abdominal organs to push directly anterior through the parietal peritoneum and transversalis fascia **in the inguinal triangle** area and into the posterior wall of the canal. Due to the larger herniation, these hernias tend not to enter the scrotum. **Direct inguinal hernias** by definition leave the abdomen **medial to the inferior epigastric vessels** because these vessels form the lateral boundary of the triangle.

COMPREHENSION QUESTIONS

[18.1] As a physician examining the inguinal region of a patient, the inguinal ligament will be a key landmark. This structure is a feature derived from which of the following?

A. Superficial fascia
B. Fascia lata of the thigh
C. Aponeurosis of the external abdominal oblique
D. Aponeurosis of the internal abdominal oblique
E. Aponeurosis of the transversus abdominis

[18.2] As you continue your examination to check for the presence of an inguinal hernia, you insert the tip of your finger into the superficial inguinal ring. This is an opening in which of the following?

A. Superficial fascia
B. Fascia lata of the thigh
C. Aponeurosis of the external abdominal oblique
D. Aponeurosis of the internal abdominal oblique
E. Aponeurosis of the transversus abdominis

[18.3] You are in the process of repairing a direct inguinal hernia. Which of the following anatomical relations will you find during surgery?

A. The hernia will enter the deep inguinal ring
B. The hernia will enter the femoral ring
C. The hernia will lie lateral to the inferior epigastric vessels
D. The hernia will lie medial to the inferior epigastric vessels
E. The hernia will lie inferior to the inguinal ligament

Answers

[18.1] **C.** The inguinal ligament is the inferior edge of the aponeurosis of the external abdominal oblique muscle.

[18.2] **C.** The superficial inguinal ring is an opening in the aponeurosis of the external abdominal oblique muscle.

[18.3] **D.** Direct inguinal hernias occur through the inguinal triangle, and the inferior epigastric vessels form the lateral boundary of this triangle. Hence, these vessels are lateral to the hernia.

ANATOMY PEARLS

 The external abdominal oblique aponeurosis forms the anterior wall and floor of the inguinal canal (inguinal ligament) and the superficial inguinal ring.

 The deep inguinal ring lies immediately lateral to the inferior epigastric vessels.

 Indirect inguinal hernias enter the deep inguinal ring (lateral to the epigastric vessels).

 Direct inguinal hernias enter the inguinal triangle (medial to the epigastric vessels).

REFERENCES

Moore KL, Dalley AF. Clinically Oriented Anatomy, 5th ed. Baltimore, MD: Lippincott Williams & Wilkins, 2006:214–20, 223–5.

Netter FH. Atlas of Human Anatomy, 4th ed. Philadelphia, PA: Saunders, 2006: plates 249, 259–60.

Snell RS. Clinical Anatomy by Regions, 8th ed. Baltimore, MD: Lippincott Williams & Wilkins, 2008:163–4, 183–5.

A 42-year-old woman is seen by her primary care physician complaining of intermittent colicky pain. She describes the pain as being right upper quadrant (RUQ), starting shortly after eating a meal, and lasting about 30 minutes. During these episodes, she says she feels bloated and nauseated. The patient also states that over the past 2 days, her stools have become very light in color, like the color of sand, and her skin has become yellow.

◆ **What is the most likely diagnosis?**

◆ **What is the anatomic basis for the clinical condition?**

ANSWERS TO CASE 19: GALLSTONES

Summary: A 42-year-old woman presents with intermittent colicky RUQ abdominal pain shortly after eating, that lasts for about 30 minutes. It is associated with bloating, nausea, and a 2-day history of acholic stools and icterus.

◆ **Most likely diagnosis:** Gallstones

◆ **Anatomical basis for condition:** Bile duct obstruction, probably by gallstones

CLINICAL CORRELATION

This middle-aged woman has the typical symptoms of biliary colic, which is intermittent crampy abdominal pain in the epigastric region of the RUQ, sometimes radiating to the right shoulder. These symptoms typically appear after meals, particularly fatty meals. The more concerning signs are the light-colored stools (acholic) and jaundice (icterus). Gallstones (cholelithiasis) are precipitated bile salts in the gallbladder, which may produce inflammation of the gallbladder (cholecystitis). Stones can pass into the cystic duct and into the common bile duct. Since the common bile duct is formed by the union of the cystic and common hepatic ducts, obstruction of the common bile duct prevents bilirubin produced in the liver from reaching the small intestines. The stools thus are lacking this pigment. As a secondary result of the obstruction, serum bilirubin is elevated, precipitated in the skin, resulting in the yellow tint. Ultrasound can often make the initial diagnosis. Removal of a common bile duct stone can be performed by upper GI endoscopy through the ampulla of Vater or surgically.

APPROACH TO GALLBLADDER

Objectives

1. Be able to describe the anatomy of the gallbladder and hepatobiliary duct system.
2. Be able to describe the clinically important anatomical relationships of the cystic and common bile ducts.

Definitions

Cholecystitis: Inflammation of the gallbladder often associated with gallstones.

DISCUSSION

The **gallbladder** is an inverted, pear-shaped, fibromuscular sac for the temporary storage and intermittent release of bile, produced in the liver. Its surface position can be approximated at the intersection of the right margin of the rectus sheath (linea semilunaris) and the right costal margin. Its anterior surface is fused to the liver between the right and quadrate lobes, and its fundus, lateral, and posterior surfaces are covered with visceral peritoneum. It is anatomically divided into fundus, body, and a neck, which is continuous with the **cystic duct.** The mucosa of the neck and cystic duct are spiral fold which acts as a valve to keep the lumen of the duct and neck open to receive bile. The gallbladder and cystic duct are supplied by the cystic artery, typically a branch of the right hepatic artery (see Figure 19-1)

The biliary duct system begins as **bile canaliculi** between hepatocytes within the liver. The canaliculi empty into microscopic interlobular bile ducts, which unite to form larger and larger ducts, eventually forming segmental and lobar ducts draining anatomical subdivisions of the liver of the same name. Ultimately, right and left hepatic ducts emerge from the liver's porta hepatis, and unite to form the **common hepatic duct** within the hepatoduadenal ligament (a portion of the lesser omentum). The cystic duct joins the common hepatic duct from the right to form the **common bile duct**. The common bile duct passes inferior within the hepatoduodenal ligament, to then pass posterior to the first part of the duodenum. It turns slightly to the right on or within the

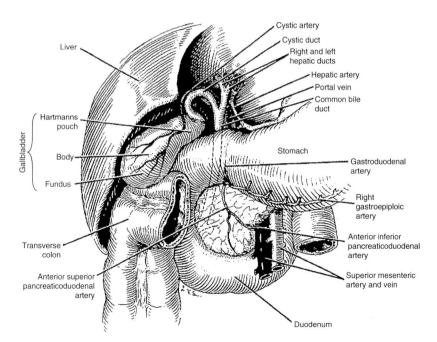

Figure 19-1. Relationships of the gallbladder. (*Reproduced, with permission, from Lindner HH. Clinical Anatomy. East Norwalk, CT: Appleton & Lange, 1989.*)

posterior surface of the pancreas. As it approaches the posteromedial wall of the duodenum, it is typically joined by the **main pancreatic duct** to form the hepatopancreatic ampulla, which opens on the major duodenal papilla.

At **the porta hepatis**, the right and left hepatic ducts are the most anterior structures. The hepatic arteries (right and left) lie posterior to the hepatic ducts, and the branches of the portal vein lie most posterior. The common hepatic duct (on the left), the cystic duct (on the right) and the inferior border of the liver (superior) form the cystohepatic **triangle of Calot**, which contains the right hepatic artery and its cystic artery branch.

Within the **hepatoduodenal ligament**, the anterior boundary of the epiploic foramen (of Winslow), the common bile duct lies to the right, the common hepatic artery lies to the left, and the portal vein lies posterior and between the duct and the artery.

COMPREHENSION QUESTIONS

[19.1] Which of the following is the correct landmark for locating the normal position of the gallbladder during a physical examination?

    A. The lowest point of the left subcostal margin
    B. The junction of the left linea semilunaris with the subcostal margin
    C. The lowest point of the right subcostal margin
    D. The junction of the right linea semilunaris with the subcostal margin
    E. The junction of the right linea semilunaris with the subcostal plane

[19.2] During a surgical procedure in which you will remove the gallbladder, you will expect its blood supply, the cystic artery, to arise from which of the following arteries?

    A. Right hepatic artery
    B. Left hepatic artery
    C. Proper hepatic artery
    D. Common hepatic artery
    E. Right gastric artery

[19.3] During the surgical procedure in the above question, your index finger is placed into the epiploic foramen. Which of the following structures would be inferior to your finger?

    A. Caudate lobe of the liver
    B. First part of the duodenum
    C. Inferior vena cava
    D. Portal vein
    E. Hepatic artery

Answers

[19.1]   **D.** The gallbladder is normally located at the junction of the right
         semilunar line with the right subcostal margin.

[19.2]   **A.** The cystic artery typically is a branch of the right hepatic artery.

[19.3]   **B.** The first part of the duodenum will lie inferior to a finger within
         the epiploic foramen.

ANATOMY PEARLS

❖ The gallbladder fossa lies between the right and quadrate lobes of
  the liver.
❖ The cystic artery is usually a branch of the right hepatic artery.
❖ The hepatic ducts are the most anterior structures at the porta
  hepatis.
❖ The bile ducts lie to the right within the hepatoduodenal ligament.

REFERENCES

Moore, K.L., Dalley, A.F. Clinically Oriented Anatomy, 5th ed. Baltimore, MD:
    Lippincott Williams & Wilkins, 2006:301–5.
Netter, F.H. Atlas of Human Anatomy, 4th ed. Philadelphia, PA: Saunders, 2006:
    294–5.
Snell, R.S. Clinical Anatomy by Regions, 8th ed. Baltimore, MD: Lippincott
    Williams & Wilkins, 2008:250–3.

A 62-year-old woman complains of the sudden onset of severe midabdominal pain that has been increasing over the past 3 hours. She has a history of myocardial ischemia and peripheral vascular disease. The patient indicates she has had nausea and vomiting. On examination, she is writhing in pain. Her abdomen has normal bowel sounds and minimal tenderness. A small amount of blood is present in the stool specimen. The electrolytes show a low bicarbonate level at 15 mEq/L, and the serum lactate level is high, which are indicative of tissue receiving insufficient oxygenation leading to tissue injury. A surgeon who is concerned about intestinal ischemia has been called to evaluate the patient.

◆ **What is the most likely diagnosis?**

◆ **What anatomical structure is likely involved?**

ANSWERS TO CASE 20: SMALL BOWEL MESENTERIC ANGINA

Summary: A 62-year-old woman with widespread atherosclerotic vascular disease complains of a 3-hour history of severe midabdominal pain accompanied by nausea and vomiting. Although writhing in pain, bowel sounds are normal, and there is minimal tenderness. Blood is present in the stool, and electrolytes show low levels of bicarbonate at 15 mEq/L and high levels of lactate; these findings are suspected as a result of lack of oxygen to intestinal tissue, leading to anaerobic metabolism. The surgeon is concerned about ischemia.

◆ **Most likely diagnosis:** Mesenteric ischemia

◆ **Anatomical structures likely involved:** Arteries that supply the small bowel, probably branches of the superior mesenteric artery (SMA)

CLINICAL CORRELATION

This elderly woman complains of sudden onset of severe midabdominal pain that is out of proportion to the physical findings. She has a history of widespread atherosclerotic vascular disease affecting the coronary arteries and peripheral vasculature. The presence of blood in the stool suggests bowel injury, and the low level of serum bicarbonate is consistent with a metabolic acidemia. Bowel ischemia or necrosis is causative. Arterial occlusion may occur from rupture of the atherosclerotic plaque or embolization from another clot. This patient's midabdominal symptoms suggest arteriography of the SMA, and the celiac artery might be diagnostic. Upon confirmation, surgical embolectomy is usually helpful. The mortality rate is high in such patients.

Although the first part of the duodenum is supplied by the superior pancreaticoduodenal artery, which receives its blood from the celiac artery, the remainder of the small intestines is supplied by branches of the SMA.

APPROACH TO VASCULAR SUPPLY TO THE BOWEL

Objectives

1. Be able to describe the general plan for the arterial blood supply to the abdominal viscera.
2. Be able to describe the anatomy and distribution of the SMA.

Definitions

Atherosclerotic vascular disease: Disease in which deposits of plaques of cholesterol and lipid form within the intima of small and medium arteries.

Angina: Pain, often severe, due to decreased blood flow to an organ such as the heart or intestines.

Superior mesenteric artery: Unpaired arterial branch of the abdominal aorta that supplies portions of the duodenum, the jejunum, ileum, cecum, appendix, ascending colon, and most of the transverse colon.

DISCUSSION

The **abdominal gastrointestinal viscera** are supplied by the **three major unpaired branches of the abdominal aorta: celiac artery (trunk), SMA, and inferior mesenteric artery (IMA).** These three arteries supply organs embryologically derived from the **foregut, midgut, and hindgut,** respectively.

The **duodenum** proximal to the entrance of the common bile duct receives its blood supply from the **superior pancreaticoduodenal artery,** a branch of the gastroduodenal artery from the celiac artery. The remainder of the small intestines is supplied by the **SMA** (Figure 20-1). The SMA arises from the abdominal aorta at the level of the lower border of L1, posterior to the neck of the pancreas. As it emerges from behind the pancreas, it passes anterior to the uncinate process of the pancreas and the third part of the duodenum and enters the **root of the mesentery.** As it enters the mesenteric root, it gives off its **inferior pancreaticoduodenal** and **middle colic arteries,** the latter to the transverse colon within its mesentery, the **transverse mesocolon.** As the SMA

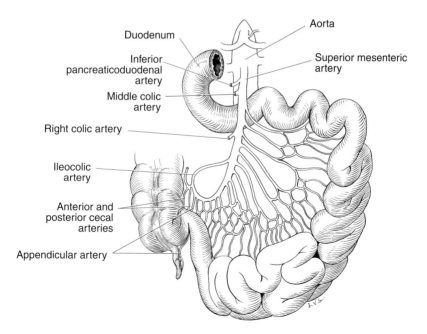

Figure 20-1. Arterial supply to the small bowel. (*Reproduced, with permission, from Lindner HH. Clinical Anatomy. East Norwalk, CT: Appleton & Lange, 1989:353.*)

descends toward the ileocolic junction, **15 to 18 intestinal branches** arise, which pass between the layers of the mesentery, and are united by increasingly complex anatomical **arcades.** The arcades closest to the mesenteric attachment to the jejunum and ileum give off increasingly shorter straight arteries (vasa recta) that enter the small intestines. Other branches of the SMA include the **right colic** to the ascending colon and the **ileocolic** to the cecum, appendix, and ascending colon.

COMPREHENSION QUESTIONS

[20.1] During a surgical procedure, you have elevated the transverse colon and note an artery in the transverse mesocolon. What is this vessel?

A. Right gastro-omental artery
B. Middle colic artery
C. Inferior pancreaticoduodenal artery
D. Right colic artery
E. Left colic artery

[20.2] During surgery you note a retroperitoneal artery crossing the right side of the posterior abdominal wall and supplying the ascending colon. Which vessel is this?

A. Middle colic artery
B. Left colic artery
C. Ileocolic artery
D. Right colic artery
E. Sigmoidal artery

[20.3] A 44-year-old accountant develops a bleeding ulcer around tax time. The gastroenterologist visualizes the ulcer in the proximal duodenum. A radiologist has been called to cannulate and embolize the artery supplying the ulcer. Which of the following arteries does the radiologist need to cannulate?

A. Celiac artery
B. SMA
C. IMA
D. Superior epigastric artery

Answers

[20.1]   **B.** The middle colic artery courses through the transverse mesocolon to supply the transverse colon.

[20.2]   **D.** The right colic artery supplies the ascending colon and is retroperitoneal.

[20.3]   **A.** The superior pancreaticoduodenal artery is a terminal branch that arises from the celiac artery.

ANATOMY PEARLS

 The SMA arises from the aorta opposite L1 posteriorly to the neck of the pancreas but crosses anterior to the third part of the duodenum.

 The celiac artery and SMA anastomose with each other through the pancreaticoduodenal arteries.

 The SMA intestinal arcades increase in complexity, but the vasa recta decrease in length from proximal to distal.

REFERENCES

Moore KL, Dalley AF. Clinically Oriented Anatomy, 5th ed. Baltimore, MD: Lippincott Williams & Wilkins, 2006:241–4, 265–7.

Netter FH. Atlas of Human Anatomy, 4th ed. Philadelphia, PA: Saunders, 2006: plates 306–7.

Snell RS. Clinical Anatomy by Regions, 8th ed. Baltimore, MD: Lippincott Williams & Wilkins, 2008:227–9, 243–4.

❖ CASE 21

An 18-year-old male college student complains of 12-hour abdominal pain that began around his umbilicus but then shifted to the right lower quadrant (RLQ) and right side. He indicates that he has been nauseous over the past several hours. His temperature is 99.4°F. On physical examination, there is mild abdominal tenderness, particularly in the RLQ, but also on the right side. The laboratory analysis of the urine is normal.

◆ **What is the most likely diagnosis?**

◆ **What accounts for the shift in location of the pain?**

ANSWERS TO CASE 21: ACUTE APPENDICITIS

Summary: An 18-year-old man complains of 12-hour abdominal pain that is initially periumbilical and then migrates to the RLQ. He has some nausea and a low-grade fever. The abdomen is tender in the RLQ and right lateral region. The urinalysis is normal.

◆ **Most likely diagnosis:** Appendicitis, possibly retrocecal.

◆ **Cause of shift in location of pain:** Pain initially irritates the visceral peritoneum, is referred to the periumbilical area, and then localized to RLQ as the appendicitis worsens and inflames the parietal peritoneum.

CLINICAL CORRELATION

This college student's complaints are suspicious for appendicitis. The appendix is a small diverticulum that arises from the cecum and is typically free in the peritoneal cavity. Not infrequently, however, it is retrocecal in location and causes right-side or flank tenderness and very few peritoneal signs. Initially, the abdominal pain is vaguely and generally located to the periumbilical region, but with time, it becomes sharper and precisely located to the RLQ. Nausea is common but presents after the onset of pain. Men and women are equally affected by appendicitis, but the diagnosis is usually more straightforward in men. A serum leukocyte count may be helpful. Ultimately, the suspicion is a clinical one, and diagnostic laparoscopy is undertaken to visualize the appendix. If appendicitis is confirmed, surgery is indicated.

APPROACH TO THE LARGE BOWEL

Objectives

1. Be able to describe the anatomy of the appendix and large intestine.
2. Be able to describe the mechanism for referred pain.
3. Be able to describe the general anatomic pattern for abdominal pain.

Definitions

Appendicitis: Inflammation of the appendix that is often associated with a fecalith, a small piece of stool that occludes the proximal appendix.
Referred pain: Pain that originates from a deep structure that is perceived at the surface of the body often at a different location.

DISCUSSION

The typical position of the appendix can be approximated at a **point (McBurney)** one-third of the way along a line drawn from the right anterior superior iliac spine to the umbilicus. The **appendix is an elongated diverticulum** that arises from the **cecum** inferior to the ileocecal junction (Figure 21-1). The three longitudinal smooth muscle bands characteristic of the cecum and colon, **the teniae coli,** can be traced inferiorly to the posteromedial origin of the appendix from the cecum. The appendix lies in the margin of a small triangular mesentery, the mesoappendix, within which the **appendicular artery** (a branch of the ileocolic artery) is also found. The posterior surface of the cecum is often covered with visceral peritoneum, creating a **retrocecal recess.** In close to 66 percent of individuals, the appendix is retrocecal in position and is found in this recess. In almost 33 percent of individuals, the appendix is free and extends inferiorly toward or over the pelvic brim. The cecum and the appendix can lie at higher or lower positions relative to McBurney point due to faulty embryonic gut rotation.

The **large intestines** are characterized by the presence **of teniae coli, haustra, omental appendices, and their large diameter.** The cecum is the pouchlike first part of the large intestines into which the ileum opens and the appendix arises. It is continuous superiorly with the ascending colon. The **ascending colon** is the shortest segment of colon, is retroperitoneal (lacks a mesentery), is continuous with the transverse colon at the right colic (hepatic) flexure, and is supplied by the ileocolic and right colic branches of the superior mesenteric artery (SMA). **The transverse colon** is the longest segment of colon, begins at the right colic flexure, and is continuous with the descending colon at the more superiorly positioned left colic (splenic) flexure. It is

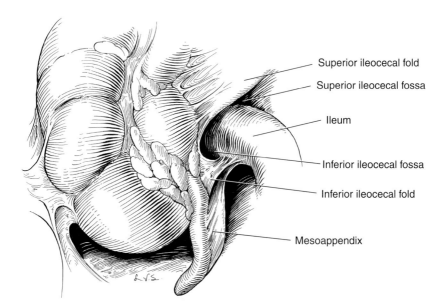

Figure 21-1. Cecal folds and fossae. (*Reproduced, with permission, from Lindner HH. Clinical Anatomy. East Norwalk, CT: Appleton & Lange, 1989:361.*)

intraperitoneal, being suspended by its mesentery, the transverse mesocolon. The **middle colic artery branch of the SMA** lies within the mesentery. The **descending colon** is retroperitoneal, continuous with the sigmoid colon near the left iliac crest, and is supplied by the **left colic artery,** a branch of the **inferior mesenteric artery (IMA).** The **sigmoid colon** is suspended by its mesentery, the sigmoid mesocolon, in which its blood supply, the several sigmoidal arteries, are found. The sigmoid colon ends at the rectosigmoid junction, which lies at the S3 vertebral level. The arteries that supply the colon are connected by continuous arterial anastomoses called the **marginal arteries.**

The **initial vague, poorly localized pain** of appendicitis results from the stretching of the **visceral peritoneum** secondary to the inflammation of the organ. The visceral afferent nerve fibers from the appendix have their cell bodies in the dorsal root ganglia and enter the spinal cord at levels T8 through T10. Sensory fibers from the umbilicus enter the spinal cord at T10. The brain misinterprets (refers) the pain from the appendix as arising from the umbilical and nearby abdominal wall. This is called referred pain. As the inflammatory process progresses, adjacent **parietal peritoneum** is typically irritated, and the pain shifts to the actual location of the appendix in the **RLQ.** The parietal peritoneum is innervated by somatic sensory nerve fibers and, when irritated, produces sharp, well-localized pain sensation. If the appendix is **retrocecal,** the parietal peritoneum of the posterior abdominal wall is irritated, resulting in **side or flank tenderness.**

Pain originating from **foregut**-derived organs and supplied by the **celiac artery** is generally perceived in the **epigastric region.** Pain from **midgut**-derived organs supplied by the **SMA** is perceived in the **periumbilical region,** and pain in the **infraumbilical** region arises from **hindgut organs (IMA).**

COMPREHENSION QUESTIONS

[21.1] You are at surgery for the removal of a suspected appendicitis, but the appendix is not visible. The appendix is likely to be which of the following?

A. Anticecal
B. Paracecal
C. Paracolic
D. Retrocecal
E. Retrocolic

[21.2] Which of the following techniques could you use to precisely locate the appendix?

A. Locate a region devoid of haustra
B. Trace the right collect artery
C. Trace the ileocolic artery
D. Trace the teniae coli on the cecum
E. Examine the pelvic cavity

[21.3] A patient experiencing infraumbilical pain is likely to have a disorder of which organ?

    A. Appendix
    B. Ascending colon
    C. Ileum
    D. Stomach
    E. Sigmoid colon

Answers

[21.1] **D.** The appendix is retrocecal in position in almost 66 percent of the population.

[21.2] **D.** The three teniae coli converge at the base of the appendix on the cecum.

[21.3] **E.** Infraumbilical pain typically arises from hindgut-derived structures such as the sigmoid colon.

ANATOMY PEARLS

 The appendix typically lies at McBurney point and is retrocecal in about 66 percent of the population.

 The SMA and IMA anastomose with each other through the marginal artery.

 The initial referred pain of appendicitis is to the periumbilical region.

REFERENCES

Moore KL, Dalley AF. Clinically Oriented Anatomy, 5th ed. Baltimore, MD: Lippincott Williams & Wilkins, 2006:271–5.

Netter FH. Atlas of Human Anatomy, 4th ed. Philadelphia, PA: Saunders, 2006: plates 281–2, 324.

Snell RS. Clinical Anatomy by Regions, 8th ed. Baltimore, MD: Lippincott Williams & Wilkins, 2008:229–32.

A 30-year-old man is admitted to the hospital for severe constant abdominal pain with nausea and vomiting since the previous day. He states the pain radiates straight to his back and feels "like it's boring a hole right through me from front to back." He reports no other medical problems, but drinks one to two six-packs of beer each weekend. He denies diarrhea or fever. The serum amylase and lipase levels are markedly elevated.

◆ **What is the most likely diagnosis?**

◆ **What is the anatomical location of the structure involved?**

ANSWERS TO CASE 22: PANCREATITIS

Summary: A 30-year-old man who drinks alcohol is admitted to the hospital for severe abdominal pain with nausea and vomiting for 24-hour duration. He states the pain radiates straight to his back. The serum amylase and lipase levels are markedly elevated.

◆ **Most likely diagnosis:** Acute pancreatitis

◆ **Anatomical location of the structure affected:** Retroperitoneal, posterior to the stomach and the lesser peritoneal sac (omental bursa)

CLINICAL CORRELATION

The pancreas is a retroperitoneal organ, posterior to the stomach and lesser sac, partly surrounded by the duodenum. It is an exocrine gland that secretes digestive enzymes and an endocrine gland that produces insulin and glucagon to regulate blood glucose levels. Noninfectious inflammation of the pancreas is most commonly caused by alcohol abuse or gallstones. The inflammation is secondary to autodigestion of the pancreatic tissue by the exocrine secretions. Marked vomiting is typical, and serum amylase or lipase levels are elevated. Immediate management includes restricting oral intake, monitoring fluid and electrolyte balance, and pain control. The pancreatitis sometimes may be so severe as to produce hemorrhage into the pancreas or pulmonary injury. These complications are associated with higher mortality rates.

APPROACH TO THE PANCREAS

Objectives

1. Be able to describe the anatomy of the pancreas and its relations to the duodenum and spleen.
2. Be able to describe the retroperitoneal relations of the pancreas.

Definitions

Pancreatitis: Inflammation of the pancreas.
Retroperitoneal: Posterior or external to the peritoneal cavity.
Omental bursa: Subdivision of the peritoneal cavity posterior to the stomach and lesser omentum.

DISCUSSION

The **pancreas is a retroperitoneal gland** that is **exocrine** (secretes digestive enzymes released into the duodenum) and **endocrine** (source of insulin and glucagon released into the bloodstream). It lies posterior to the omental bursa (lesser sac). The gland is anatomically divided into **head, neck, body, and tail** regions and is diagonally placed across the posterior abdominal wall (Figure 22-1). The head of the pancreas lies within the curve of the second and third parts of the duodenum, and its inferior portion forms a hook-like uncinate process that lies posterior to the superior mesenteric vessels. The neck lies at the L1 vertebral level, with the pylorus of the stomach immediately superior. The portal vein is formed posteriorly by the union of the splenic vein and superior mesenteric vein (SMV). The body of the gland passes superiorly to the left, with the tortuous splenic artery along its superior border. The short tail of the pancreas lies within the splenorenal ligament and may contact the hilum of the spleen (Table 22-1).

The exocrine pancreas is drained by a **main pancreatic duct,** which begins in the tail, and passes to the right through the body, neck, and inferior portion of the head. The **duct pierces the wall of the second part of the duodenum** in close association with the **common bile duct,** with which it typically unites to form the **hepatopancreatic ampulla,** which in turn opens through the major **duodenal papilla.** Several smooth muscle sphincters surround these ducts, which may enter the duodenum separately at the papilla. The superior portion of the head is drained by an accessory pancreatic duct that usually joins the main duct but may drain separately into the duodenum at the minor duodenal papilla. The head of the pancreas receives its arterial blood supply primarily from superior and inferior **pancreaticoduodenal arteries** from the

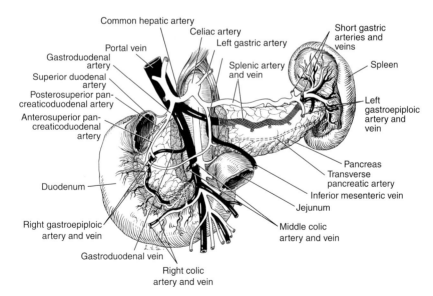

Figure 22-1. The pancreas and its blood supply. (*Reproduced, with permission, from Lindner HH. Clinical Anatomy. East Norwalk, CT: Appleton & Lange, 1989:346.*)

Table 22-1
STRUCTURES POSTERIOR TO THE PANCREAS

HEAD	NECK	BODY	TAIL
IVC	SMA and SMV	Aorta	Splenic vein
Right renal vessels	Splenic vein	SMA	
Left renal vein	Portal vein (formed)	Splenic vein	
		Left kidney and suprarenal gland	
		Left renal vessels	

celiac and superior mesenteric artery (SMA), respectively, whereas the neck, body, and tail receive branches from the splenic artery.

The **duodenum** is the first, shortest, widest, and least mobile portion of the small intestine. It is anatomically subdivided into four parts, and its C-shaped configuration is intimately related to the pancreas. The superior or first part is the posteriorly directed continuation of the pylorus of the stomach, and it lies at the L1 vertebral level. Its first portion or ampulla (clinically, the duodenal cap) is intraperitoneal, within the hepatoduodenal ligament. The remainder is retroperitoneal. The descending or second part is retroperitoneal, lies opposite L1, L2, and L3, and receives the pancreatic and bile ducts (hepatopancreatic ampulla) at the major duodenal papilla on its posteromedial wall. The horizontal or third part is also retroperitoneal, passes to the left, and crosses L3. The SMA and SMV cross this part of the duodenum anteriorly. The ascending or fourth part lies on the left side of the L3 and L2 vertebrae and is retroperitoneal, except perhaps for the last few millimeters as it becomes continuous with the jejunum at the duodenojejunal junction, indicated anatomically by the **suspensory ligament of Treitz.** The clinically important relations of the duodenum are listed in Table 22-2. The **duodenum** is supplied by **superior and inferior pancreaticoduodenal arteries** from the **celiac artery and SMA, respectively.**

The **spleen** is the largest lymph organ of the body and functions as if it were a lymph node for the circulatory system. It is intraperitoneal, being suspended in the left upper quadrant by the **gastrosplenic and splenorenal ligaments** (subdivisions of the greater omentum). It lies parallel to the 10th rib and overlaps the 9th and 11th ribs. It has a convex diaphragmatic surface and concave hilum, where the ligaments attach. The **splenic artery** (a major branch of the celiac artery) enters, and the splenic vein exits the spleen through the hilum and is within the splenorenal ligament in addition to the tail of the pancreas.

Table 22-2

ANATOMICAL RELATIONS OF THE DUODENUM

	ANTERIOR	POSTERIOR	MEDIAL	SUPERIOR
Superior or first part	Gallblader	Bile duct		Epiploic foramen
	Quadrate lobe of liver	Gastroduodenal artery		
		Portal vein		
		IVC		
Descending or second part	Transverse mesocolon	Hilum right kidney	Head of pancreas	
	Transverse colon	Renal vessels and pelvis	Bile and pancreatic ducts	
	Small intestines	Right ureter		
		Right psoas muscle		
Horizontal or third part	SMA and SMV	IVC and aorta		Head and uncinate process of pancreas
	Small intestines	Right ureter		SMA and SMV
		Right psoas muscle		
Ascending or fourth part	Root of mesentery	Aorta, left side	Head of pancreas	Body of pancreas
	Small intestines	Left psoas muscle		

COMPREHENSION QUESTIONS

[22.1] You are at surgery and are about to mobilize the second portion of the duodenum and the head of the pancreas. You note an artery and vein passing anteriorly to the uncinate process of the pancreas and the third portion of the duodenum. Which vessels are these?

A. SMA and SMV
B. Inferior mesenteric artery and vein
C. Gastroduodenal artery and vein
D. Superior pancreaticoduodenal artery and vein
E. Middle colic artery and vein

[22.2] As you proceed to elevate the duodenum and pancreas, you note two veins posterior to the neck of the pancreas uniting to form a large vein that passes superiorly. Which large vein has been formed?

A. Splenic vein
B. IVC
C. Portal vein
D. Right gastric vein
E. Middle colic vein

[22.3] As you continue, you also note a large, tortuous artery passing to the left along the superior border of the pancreas. This is likely to be which of the following?

A. Left renal artery
B. IMA
C. Splenic artery
D. Left gastroomental artery
E. Left colic artery

Answers

[22.1]   **A.** The SMA and SMV emerge from between the head and uncinate process of the pancreas to cross the uncinate process and the third portion of the duodenum.

[22.2]   **C.** The portal vein is formed by the union of the superior mesenteric and splenic veins posterior to the neck of the pancreas.

[22.3]   **C.** The splenic artery, the most tortuous artery of the body, is located along the superior border of the pancreas as it passes to the left toward the spleen.

ANATOMY PEARLS

 The pancreas is retroperitoneal, posterior to the omental bursa.

 The splenic artery passes along the superior border of the pancreas, whereas the splenic vein lies posterior.

The portal vein is formed posterior to the neck of the pancreas.

 The hepatoduodenal papilla (bile and pancreatic ducts) opens onto the major duodenal papilla on the posteromedial wall of the second part of the duodenum.

 The second part of the duodenum is related to the right kidney hilum, pelvis and ureter, and renal vessels posteriorly.

The third part of the duodenum is crossed anteriorly by the SMA and SMV.

REFERENCES

Moore KL, Dalley AF. Clinically Oriented Anatomy, 5th ed. Baltimore, MD: Lippincott Williams & Wilkins, 2006:286–9.

Netter FH. Atlas of Human Anatomy, 4th ed. Philadelphia, PA: Saunders, 2006: plates 298, 301.

Snell RS. Clinical Anatomy by Regions, 8th ed. Baltimore, MD: Lippincott Williams & Wilkins, 2008:256–8.

A 38-year-old man comes into the emergency department presenting with fatigue and abdominal swelling. For several months, he has noticed that his abdomen has been growing larger and that his skin has turned yellow. He denies any medical problems but admits to drinking alcohol almost every day. On examination, his skin clearly has a yellow hue indicative of icterus. His palms have some redness. His abdomen is markedly distended and tense, and a fluid wave is present. On the surface of the abdomen there are prominent vascular markings.

◆ **What is the most likely diagnosis?**

◆ **What organs are likely to be affected?**

ANSWERS TO CASE 23: CIRRHOSIS

Summary: A 38-year-old icteric man who abuses alcohol enters the emergency department for fatigue and abdominal "swelling." He has palmar erythema and abdominal distention with a positive fluid wave and prominent vascular markings.

◆ **Most likely diagnosis:** Alcoholic cirrhosis with portal hypertension

◆ **Organs likely affected:** Liver and those drained by the portal venous system

CLINICAL CORRELATION

This patient abuses alcohol and has manifestations of end-stage liver disease (cirrhosis). Cirrhosis results in severe fibrotic scarring of the liver, which decreases blood flow through the organ. Hypertension in the portal venous system is the result, with collateral venous flow, especially in organs having venous drainage by the portal and vena caval systems, such as the abdominal surface, and the esophagus. The spleen is frequently enlarged, and the ascites, fluid within the peritoneal cavity, is due to liver insufficiency. Death may ensue due to bleeding from esophageal varices or bacterial peritonitis of the ascitic fluid. Marked hepatic insufficiency is another complication.

APPROACH TO THE LIVER

Objectives

1. Be able to describe the anatomy of the liver and its unique blood supply.
2. Be able to draw the anatomy of the portal venous system and the clinically important sites of anastomosis with the vena caval system.

Definitions

Cirrhosis: Disease of progressive degeneration of the liver in which damage to the liver cells results in nodular regeneration, fibrosis, and impedance.

Portacaval anastomosis: Communication between tributaries of the portal venous system and the systemic venous system.

Portal hypertension: Increased pressure in the portal venous system with resultant reverse flow, typically due to obstructed venous flow through the liver, as in cirrhosis.

Fluid wave: Maneuver during physical examination in which tapping on one side of the abdomen leads to the sensation of force traveling to the other side of the abdomen, suggesting the presence of intra-abdominal fluid.

DISCUSSION

The **liver, the largest internal organ,** has a **convex diaphragmatic surface** that conforms to the curvature of the diaphragm and an **irregular concave visceral surface.** The liver is covered with visceral peritoneum over most of its surface and is suspended by several mesenteric structures called ligaments. The **falciform ligament** (with the **round ligament of the liver,** the adult remnant of the umbilical vein, in its free margin) is reflected onto the anterior abdominal wall and divides the liver into apparent right and left anatomical lobes. As the falciform ligament passes onto the superior surface of the liver, the two layers of peritoneum diverge to the right and to the left, creating the anterior layers of the **coronary ligaments.** These pass to the right and to the left to the extremes of the superior liver surface, turn back on themselves (creating the **triangular ligaments**), and turn posteriorly to form the posterior layers of the coronary ligaments. In this manner, an area devoid of visceral peritoneum is created, the **bare area of the liver.** The posterior layers of the coronary ligaments converge to form the **lesser omentum,** which passes from the visceral surface of the liver to the lesser curvature of the stomach (**hepatogastric ligament**) and the first part of the duodenum (**hepatoduodenal ligament**).

The **liver** is divided anatomically into **four lobes by external landmarks** and is delineated on the visceral surface by fissures and fossae, which **form an "H."** (See Figure 23-1.) The **right side of the H** is formed by **fossae for the gallbladder and the IVC,** and the **right lobe lies to the right** of these structures. The **left side of the H** is formed by the **fissure for the round ligament**

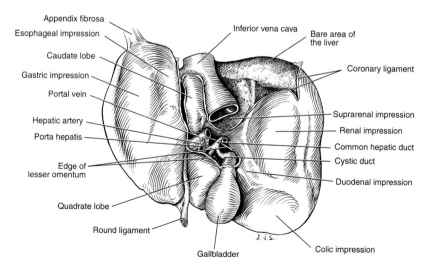

Figure 23-1. The visceral surface of the liver. (*Reproduced, with permission, from Lindner HH. Clinical Anatomy. East Norwalk, CT: Appleton & Lange, 1989:399.*)

and the ligamentum venosum (adult remnant of the ductus venosus); the **left lobe is to the left of this fissure.** The **crossbar of the H is the porta hepatis through which the hepatic artery, portal vein, and nerves** enter the liver and the **bile ducts and lymphatics exit.** The crossbar subdivides the central portion into **quadrate** and **caudate lobes.** Functionally, the right portal lobe lies to the right of the fossae of the gallbladder, IVC, and a portion of the caudate lobe. The left portal lobe is the left anatomical lobe, quadrate lobe, and the remainder of the caudate lobe. The portal lobes are supplied by lobar branches of the hepatic artery, portal vein, and bile ducts. Although lacking external landmarks, the portal lobes are further divided functionally into hepatic segments.

The liver receives a **dual blood supply;** approximately **30 percent of the blood entering the organ is from the hepatic artery, and 70 percent is from the portal vein.** The proper hepatic artery is a branch of the common hepatic artery, one of the three major branches of the celiac artery. As it approaches the liver, it divides into right and left hepatic branches that enter the liver and divide into lobar, segmental, and smaller branches. Eventually blood reaches the arterioles in the portal areas at the periphery of the hepatic lobules and, after providing oxygen and nutrients to the parenchyma, drain into the hepatic sinusoids. The majority of blood entering the liver is venous blood rich in nutrients and molecules absorbed by the gastrointestinal organs. Intrahepatic branches of the portal vein follow the arteries to the portal areas, where portal venules empty into the sinusoids from which molecules are extracted and added. Sinusoidal blood flows to the central vein of each lobule from which increasingly larger veins are formed until typically three hepatic veins exit the liver to join the IVC (Figure 23-2).

The **portal venous system** arises from the capillary beds within the abdominal organs supplied by the **celiac artery, superior mesenteric artery (SMA), and inferior mesenteric artery (IMA)** and blood will flow to and through the liver for metabolism of its contained molecules. Veins from these organs, for the most part, accompany arteries of the same name. The **portal vein itself is formed by the union of the splenic vein and SMV posterior to the neck of the pancreas.** This short, wide vein ascends within the hepatoduodenal ligament, posterior to the bile duct and hepatic artery, and enters the liver through the porta hepatis. Typically, the IMV drains its blood into the splenic vein.

Portacaval (systemic) venous anastomoses occur at sites where blood may ultimately **drain into the portal system and/or the vena caval system.** If venous flow through the portal system is prevented by liver disease, for example, the absence of valves within the portal system veins allows reverse flow. This dilates the smaller veins and blood is drained by veins emptying into the vena cavae. This occurs at several sites and may produce clinical signs or symptoms (Table 23-1).

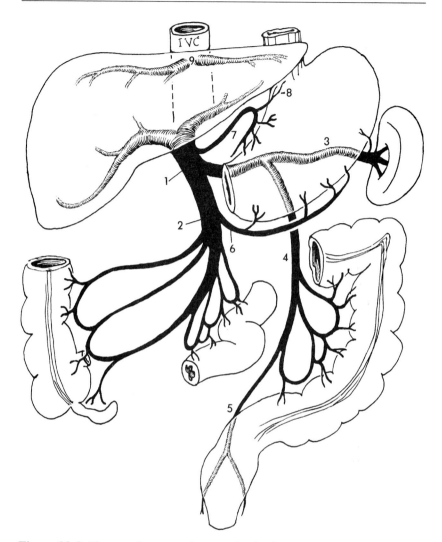

Figure 23-2. The portal system: 1 = portal vein, 2 = superior mesenteric vein, 3 = splenic vein, 4 = inferior mesenteric vein, 5 = superior rectal vein, 6 = right gastroepiploic vein, 7 = left gastric vein, 8 = esophageal vein, 9 = hepatic veins. (*Reproduced, with permission, from the University of Texas Health Science Center Houston Medical School.*)

Table 23-1

SITES OF PORTAL-CAVAL VENOUS ANASTOMOSES

	PORTAL VENOUS DRAINAGE	VENA CAVA VENOUS DRAINAGE	SIGN/SYMPTOM
Esophagus	Left gastric vein	Hemiazygous vein	Esophageal varices, bleeding
Rectum	Superior rectal vein	Inferior rectal vein	Hemorrhoids
Anterior abdominal wall	Paraumbilical vein	Intercostal vein	Caput medusa
Retroperitoneal	Duodenal, pancreatic, right and left colic veins	Lumbar vein	Intestinal bleeding

COMPREHENSION QUESTIONS

[23.1] You are examining the liver during a surgical procedure. The gallbladder will be found in its fossa between which two anatomical lobes?

A. Quadrate and left lobes
B. Quadrate and caudate lobes
C. Right and quadrate lobes
D. Caudate and right lobes
E. Caudate and left lobes

[23.2] If you ligated the right hepatic artery, the arterial supply to which of the following portions of the liver would *remain* intact?

A. Right lobe only
B. Right and quadrate lobes
C. Left lobe only
D. Left and quadrate lobes only
E. Left, quadrate, and a portion of the caudate lobe

[23.3] Your patient who had cirrhosis has symptoms of esophageal varices. This is due to dilatation of the anastomosis between which of the following pairs of veins?

A. Left gastric and the azygous veins
B. Right gastric and the azygous veins
C. Right gastric and the hemiazygous
D. Left gastric and the hemiazygous
E. Azygous and the hemiazygous

Answers

[23.1]   **C.** The gallbladder is located between the right lobe and the quadrate lobe.

[23.2]   **E.** The left hepatic artery supplies the left and quadrate lobes and a portion of the caudate lobe.

[23.3]   **D.** Esophageal veins drain to the left gastric and the hemiazygous veins.

ANATOMY PEARLS

 The left anatomical lobe, quadrate lobe, and a portion of the caudate lobe constitute the left portal lobe.

 Hemorrhage from the liver can be controlled by clamping the hepatoduodenal ligament (Pringle maneuver), which contains the hepatic artery and portal vein.

 The portal vein drains blood from organs supplied by the celiac artery, SMA, and IMA.

 Esophageal varices with bleeding is the most clinically significant symptom of portal hypertension.

REFERENCES

Moore KL, Dalley AF. Clinically Oriented Anatomy, 5th ed. Baltimore, MD: Lippincott Williams & Wilkins, 2006:289–300.

Netter FH. Atlas of Human Anatomy, 4th ed. Philadelphia, PA: Saunders, 2006: plates 287–8, 311–12.

Snell RS. Clinical Anatomy by Regions, 8th ed. Baltimore, MD: Lippincott Williams & Wilkins, 2008:246–9.

A 42-year-old male executive complains of abdominal pain that began about 6 months previously, is constant in nature especially after meals, and located in the upper midabdomen superior to the umbilicus. He also reports some "heartburn" that has been occurring during the previous year. He has been under a lot of job-related stress and has been self-medicating himself with over-the-counter antacids, with some relief. He states his stools have changed in color over the previous 2 months and now are intermittently dark and tarry in consistency. The physician tests the patient's stool and finds occult blood.

◆ **What is the most likely diagnosis?**

◆ **What organs are likely to be affected?**

ANSWERS TO CASE 24: PEPTIC ULCER DISEASE

Summary: A 42-year-old stressed-out male executive has a 6-month history of constant upper abdominal pain and heartburn for the past year that was relieved by over-the-counter antacids. His stools have become dark and tarry, which at examination, have occult blood.

◆ **Most likely diagnosis:** Peptic ulcer disease

◆ **Organs likely affected:** Stomach or duodenum

CLINICAL CORRELATION

This patient has a history typical for peptic ulcer disease, that is, constant mid-epigastric pain after meals. The patient also has symptoms consistent with gastroesophageal reflux disease. The dark and tarry stools reflect blood in the stools, that is, hemoglobin has been converted to melena. This is suggestive of an upper gastrointestinal bleeding disorder. The next step would be an upper endoscopy to visualize the suspected ulcer. If the stomach is the site, a biopsy is usually performed to assess concurrent malignancy. Treatment includes a histamine-blocking agent, proton pump inhibitor, and antibiotic therapy. The bacterium *Helicobacter pylori* has been implicated in most cases of peptic ulcer disease. If an ulcer occurs in the duodenum, the posterior wall of the ampulla of the duodenum (duodenal cap) is the usual site. The gastroduodenal artery lies posterior to the duodenum at this point and is at risk in the event of ulcer perforation.

APPROACH TO THE STOMACH

Objectives

1. Be able to describe the anatomy of the stomach.
2. Be able to describe the anatomy of the celiac artery (trunk).

Definitions

Gastroesophageal reflux disease: Condition in which gastric contents are regurgitated into the esophagus.

Peptic ulcer disease: A lesion of the gastric or duodenal mucosa with inflammation.

Helicobacter pylori: Bacterium found in the mucosa of humans and associated with peptic ulcer disease.

Endoscopy: Procedure by which the interiors of hollow organs are examined with a flexible instrument called an endoscope.

DISCUSSION

The **stomach,** the **first major gastrointestinal organ in which digestion occurs, produces digestive enzymes and hydrochloric acid (HCl).** This continuation of the esophagus is a large, intraperitoneal, saccular organ that is suspended by the mesentery-like greater and lesser omenta. The stomach is divided anatomically into a **cardia, fundus, body, and pylorus (pyloric antrum and canal with sphincter)** and has **greater and lesser curvatures.** The **greater omentum** attaches to the greater curvature and drapes inferiorly to form a double-layered apron anterior to the abdominal cavity contents. It fuses superiorly with the transverse mesocolon. The greater omentum is subdivided into gastrocolic, gastrosplenic, splenorenal, and gastrophrenic ligament portions. The **lesser omentum** is attached to the lesser curvature and first part of the duodenum and extends to the visceral surface of the liver. With the stomach, it forms the anterior boundary of the omental bursa (lesser sac). The lesser omentum is divided into hepatogastric and hepatoduodenal ligaments, with the latter forming the anterior boundary of the **epiploic foramen (of Winslow;** Figure 24-1).

The stomach is richly supplied by **five sets of arteries,** all of which are branches of the **celiac artery (trunk).** The celiac artery arises from the

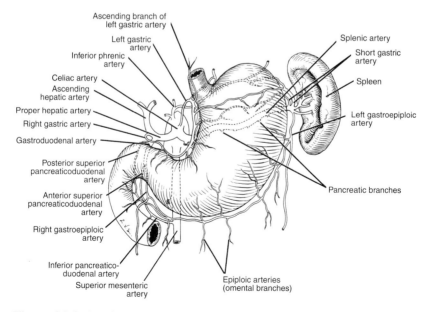

Figure 24-1. Arterial supply to the stomach. (*Reproduced, with permission, from Lindner HH. Clinical Anatomy. East Norwalk, CT: Appleton & Lange, 1989:334.*)

abdominal aorta opposite the upper portion of L1. This very short artery quickly divides into three branches. The smallest is the **left gastric artery,** which ascends toward the gastroesophageal junction at the lesser curvature. After sending small branches to the esophagus, it curves inferiorly within the lesser omentum, parallel to the lesser curvature, to which numerous **gastric branches** are provided. The **splenic artery is a large, tortuous branch** of the celiac that passes to the left, along the superior margin of the pancreas, to reach the spleen. It sends several branches to the pancreas and, as it approaches the spleen, gives off two sets of arteries to the stomach. Passing superiorly, **four to five small short gastric arteries** ascend within the gastrosplenic ligament to supply the fundus. Also near the spleen, the **left gastro-omental (epiploic) artery** arises from the splenic artery and passes inferiorly within the gastrosplenic and gastrocolic ligaments. It courses parallel to the greater curvature, to which it sends numerous branches. The last branch of the celiac is the **common hepatic artery,** which passes to the right to enter the hepatoduodenal ligament. The common hepatic divides into two branches. The proper hepatic artery ascends toward the liver within the hepatoduodenal ligament to supply the liver and gallbladder. The **right gastric artery** typically arises from the proper hepatic, descends to the gastroduodenal junction, curves superiorly and parallel to the lesser curvature, sends gastric branches to the stomach, and **anastomoses with the left gastric artery.** The other branch of the common hepatic artery is the **gastroduodenal artery,** which descends posterior to the first part of the duodenum and then divides into the pancreaticoduodenal and right gastro-omental arteries. This latter vessel lies within the gastrocolic ligament and courses to the left parallel to the greater curvature, to which gastric branches are sent. It anastomoses with the left gastro-omental along the greater curvature.

COMPREHENSION QUESTIONS

[24.1] Gastric contents exiting a posterior perforation of the stomach wall will accumulate in which of the following?

A. The left paracolic gutter
B. The left paravertebral gutter
C. The right paravertebral gutter
D. The omental bursa
E. The hepatorenal recess

[24.2] Ligation of the common hepatic artery will eliminate the gastric blood supply through which of the following arteries?

A. Left gastric and short gastric arteries
B. Short gastric and right gastro-omental arteries
C. Right gastro-omental and right gastric arteries
D. Right gastric and left gastric arteries
E. Left gastric and left gastro-omental arteries

[24.3] A surgical incision through the fundus of the stomach would require you to clamp which of the following?

    A. Right gastric artery

    B. Left gastric artery

    C. Right gastro-omental artery

    D. Left gastro-omental artery

    E. Short gastric arteries

Answers

[24.1] **D.** The omental bursa lies immediately posteriorly to the stomach.

[24.2] **C.** Blood flow through the right gastric and right gastro-omental arteries would be lost with ligation of the common hepatic artery.

[24.3] **E.** The short gastric arteries supply the fundus of the stomach.

> ## ANATOMY PEARLS
>
> ❖ The relatively fixed points of the stomach are the gastroesophageal junction and the pylorus, which lie at vertebral levels T11 and L1, respectively.
> ❖ The stomach is supplied by all three branches of the celiac artery.
> ❖ The short gastric and left gastro-omental arteries lie within the gastrosplenic ligament and are at risk in a splenectomy.

REFERENCES

    Moore KL, Dalley AF. Clinically Oriented Anatomy, 5th ed. Baltimore, MD: Lippincott Williams & Wilkins, 2006:248–59.

    Netter FH. Atlas of Human Anatomy, 4th ed. Philadelphia, PA: Saunders, 2006: plates 272, 275, 300.

    Snell RS. Clinical Anatomy by Regions, 8th ed. Baltimore, MD: Lippincott Williams & Wilkins, 2008:219–24.

A 55-year-old male is admitted to the hospital for a suspected kidney infection. He is placed on intravenous antibiotic therapy but continues to have a temperature of 103°F after 3 days of therapy. The urine culture grows *Escherichia coli*, which is sensitive to the antibiotics being used. On examination, he appears ill and has marked left flank tenderness. Ultrasound depicts an abnormal collection of fluid around the left kidney.

◆ **What is the most likely diagnosis?**

◆ **What anatomical structure is involved?**

ANSWERS TO CASE 25: PERINEPHRIC ABSCESS

Summary: A 55-year-old male continues with high fever and flank pain despite 3 days of broad-spectrum intravenous antibiotic therapy. The urine isolate of *E. coli* demonstrates in vitro sensitivity to the antibiotics used. Renal ultrasound shows fluid around the left kidney.

◆ **Most likely diagnosis:** Perinephric abscess

◆ **Anatomical structure involved:** Kidney and anatomically related structures

CLINICAL CORRELATION

This 55-year-old male who is suspected of having pyelonephritis is not improving despite appropriate antibiotic therapy. Pyelonephritis is an infection of the kidney parenchyma usually caused by an ascending infection of bacteria that advances from the urethra to bladder to ureters and then to the kidney. Kidney infection usually manifests as fever, flank tenderness, white cells in the urine, and serum leukocytosis. After 48 to 72 hours, one would expect decreases in fever and flank tenderness. *E. coli* is isolated, which is the bacterium that most often causes urinary tract infection. The ultrasound examination is performed to rule out complications of pyelonephritis. The two most common complications would be a nephrolithiasis or ureterolithiasis (kidney stone) and perinephric abscess. Intervention is required before improvement is seen. The abscess must be drained, usually by placement of a percutaneous catheter under radiologic guidance.

APPROACH TO THE KIDNEYS

Objectives

1. Be able to describe the anatomy of the kidneys, their fascial coverings, and blood supply.
2. Be aware of the structures next to the kidneys and their relations.

Definitions

Perinephric abscess: Collection of pus in the tissues surrounding the kidney.
Pyelonephritis: Usually a bacterial inflammation of the renal tissue, the calyces, or renal pelvis.
Nephrolithiasis: Presence of renal calculi or stones.

DISCUSSION

The **kidneys are paired retroperitoneal organs** that are located in the **paravertebral gutters.** The **left kidney lies slightly higher than the right,** its hilum is at the **level of L1,** and its superior and inferior poles are at the 11th rib and L3, respectively. The hilum of the **right kidney lies at the level of the disc between L1 and L2,** and its inferior pole is nearly 1 to 2 cm superior to the iliac crest. Each kidney is an encapsulated solid organ, with an outer cortex and an inner medulla, with the latter arranged in renal pyramids. The hilum of each kidney leads to a space, the renal sinus, which contains fat, branches of the renal vessels, and the urine-collecting structures (minor and major calyces and renal pelvis). Within the sinus, the apex of the 6 to 12 renal pyramids is cupped by a minor calyx, which collects the urine produced. Typically two to three minor calyces unite to form a major calyx, and two to three major calyces form the renal pelvis. The renal pelvis is continuous with the ureter at the inferior margin of the hilum (see Case 32 for the anatomy of the ureter).

Four muscles are related to each kidney posteriorly: the diaphragm superiorly and the transverses abdominis, quadratus lumborum, and psoas muscles inferiorly, from lateral to medial. The **suprarenal glands and colon contact both kidneys anteriorly.** The **duodenum and liver also contact the right kidney anteriorly,** and the **stomach, pancreas, and spleen are related to the anterior left kidney.**

Each **kidney and suprarenal gland is encased in a renal (Gerota) fascia** (Figure 25-1), which helps to maintain the position of the kidney. The renal fascia fuses with the fascia of the psoas muscle posteriorly and with the adventitia

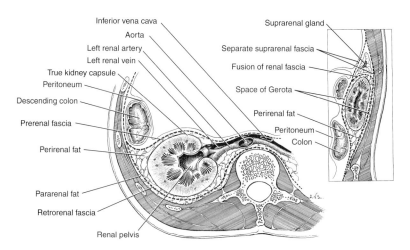

Figure 25-1. The left kidney and surrounding fascia. (*Reproduced, with permission, from Lindner HH. Clinical Anatomy. East Norwalk, CT:Appleton & Lange, 1989:444.*)

of the renal vessels anteriorly. Within the renal fascia is an accumulation of fat known as **perirenal fat,** which is continuous with the fat within the renal sinus. **Pararenal fat** surrounds each kidney external to the renal fascia. Pararenal fat is thick posterior to the kidney, but thin anteriorly between the renal fascia and parietal peritoneum.

Each kidney is supplied by a renal artery that arises from the aorta near vertebral level L2. As each artery nears the renal pelvis, it typically divides into five segmental arteries that enter the hilum to supply segments of renal tissue. The **right renal artery is the longer artery,** and **both renal arteries lie posterior to the renal veins** when entering the hilum. The renal veins exit the hilum anterior to the arteries, and the left vein is longer and crosses the midline. **Both renal veins drain into the IVC.** The **left renal vein is unique in that the inferior phrenic, suprarenal, and gonadal veins drain into it** (the IVC receives these veins on the right side).

COMPREHENSION QUESTIONS

[25.1] During the removal of a patient's kidney, you would observe which of the following as being most anterior within the renal sinus?

   A. Renal arteries
   B. Renal vein
   C. Major calyx
   D. Minor calyx
   E. Renal pelvis

[25.2] You wish to examine the hilum of the right kidney during surgery. Which of the following structures must be elevated and reflected to do so?

   A. Stomach
   B. Suprarenal gland
   C. Ascending colon
   D. Duodenum
   E. Liver

[25.3] To elevate the kidney within the renal fascia and the perirenal fat, the renal fascia must be reflected or incised from the fascia of which of the following muscles?

   A. Diaphragm
   B. Psoas muscle
   C. Quadratus lumborum muscle
   D. Transverses abdominis muscle
   E. Iliacus muscle

Answers

[25.1]   **B.** The renal veins lie most anterior within the renal sinus.
[25.2]   **D.** The duodenum lies immediately anteriorly to the hilum of the right kidney.
[25.3]   **B.** The renal fascia is fused posteriorly to the fascia of the psoas muscle.

ANATOMY PEARLS

❖ The hilum of the left kidney lies at the level of L1.
❖ In the renal sinus, the renal vessels lie anterior to the renal pelvis, with the renal vein being the most anterior.
❖ The left renal vein receives the inferior phrenic, suprarenal, and gonadal vessels.

REFERENCES

Moore KL, Dalley AF. Clinically Oriented Anatomy, 5th ed. Baltimore, MD: Lippincott Williams & Wilkins, 2006:311–17.
Netter FH. Atlas of Human Anatomy, 4th ed. Philadelphia, PA: Saunders, 2006: plates 329, 332, 342.
Snell RS. Clinical Anatomy by Regions, 8th ed. Baltimore, MD: Lippincott Williams & Wilkins, 2008:260–5.

An 18-year-old female presents with increasing hair growth on her face and chest, deepening of her voice, and acne over the past year. She has no history of other medical problems. On examination, she has acne, abnormal male pattern balding, and enlargement of her clitoris. The pelvic examination is normal including the ovaries. Blood tests show that the serum testosterone levels are normal, but that the level of dihydroepiandrostenedione sulfate, an adrenal androgen, is markedly elevated.

◆ **What is the most likely diagnosis?**

ANSWER TO CASE 26: SUPRARENAL GLAND TUMOR

Summary: An 18-year-old female is seen for increasing hirsutism, deepening voice, and acne over the past year. She has no other medical problems. On examination she displays acne, hirsutism, temporal balding, and clitoromegaly. The pelvic examination, including the ovaries, is normal. The testosterone level is normal, and the level of dihydroepiandrostenedione sulfate is markedly elevated.

◆   **Most likely diagnosis:** Suprarenal (adrenal) gland tumor

CLINICAL CORRELATION

This young female has more than hirsutism, which is increased hair growth. She also has virilism, or the effects of androgens on the skin, voice, and clitoris. The hyperandrogenism seems to be of acute onset, which is consistent with an androgen-secreting tumor. The two possibilities include an ovarian tumor, usually Sertoli-Leydig cell tumor, or an adrenal tumor. Because the pelvic examination and testosterone levels are normal, an ovarian etiology is less likely. Moreover, the high level of dihydroepiandrostenedione sulfate almost establishes the suprarenal (adrenal) gland as the cause. The next step would be a CT or MRI scan of the suprarenal glands to determine the exact location of the tumor. Usually surgery is indicated. Another cause of hirsutism is polycystic ovarian syndrome, which includes hirsutism, obesity, anovulation, and irregular menses. Cushing syndrome or disease presents strong cortisol effects, such as buffalo hump, abdominal striae, easy bruising, and central obesity.

APPROACH TO THE SUPRARENAL GLANDS

Objectives

1.   Be able to describe the anatomy of the suprarenal glands.
2.   Be able to describe the general pattern of lymphatic drainage of the abdomen.

Definitions

Virilism: Presence of mature male characteristics in a female or a prepubescent male.

Clitoromegaly: Enlargement of the clitoris.

Dihydroepiandrostenedione (DHEA): Male steroid hormone secreted by the testis, ovary, or adrenal cortex.

DISCUSSION

The **paired suprarenal glands are retroperitoneal endocrine glands** composed of an **outer cortex that secretes corticosteroid and androgen steroid hormones** and an **inner medulla (derived from neural crest cells) that secretes the catecholamines, epinephrine and norepinephrine.** Each gland **sits on the superior pole of each kidney, enclosed within the renal fascia,** and, hence, embedded in the perirenal fat. The **right suprarenal gland** is somewhat triangular and is closely related to the IVC, liver, and diaphragm. The **left gland is shaped like a comma** and related to the spleen, pancreas, stomach, and diaphragm. The suprarenal glands receive their blood supply from multiple small branches that arise from the inferior phrenic, aorta, and renal arteries. Each gland is drained by a single suprarenal vein that terminates in the IVC on the right, and the renal vein on the left.

The **lymphatic drainage of the abdomen** is diagrammatically summarized in Figure 26-1. In general, the lymphatic drainage of abdominal organs reversely follows their arterial blood supply. Thus the **lymph drainage from organs supplied by the SMA will be to the superior mesenteric nodes** by way of vessels and other node groups located along the branches of the SMA. If a **"final common pathway" for lymph drainage** in the abdomen could be named, it would be the **lumbar (aortic) lymph nodes,** and lymph from these nodes drains to the **cisterna chili and thoracic duct.** Lymph from the **suprarenal glands drains into the lumbar lymph nodes.** Figure 26-1 shows that the lymphatics from the gonads also drain to the upper lumbar nodes as the gonadal vessels arise in the upper abdomen (reflecting the site of their embryologic origin). Note also that the **pectinate line in the anal canal is a watershed with regard to lymphatic drainage.** The anal canal and rectum **superior to this line have their lymph drained to iliac nodes; inferior to this line, lymph drains to inguinal nodes.**

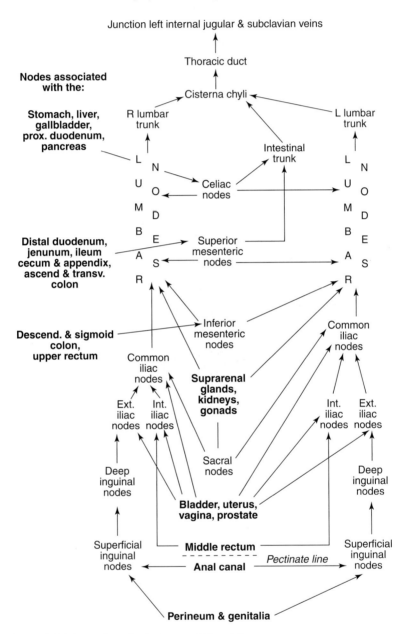

Figure 26-1. Lymph node drainage of the abdomen.

COMPREHENSION QUESTIONS

[26.1] As a surgeon about to remove the right adrenal gland, you examine the blood supply of the right adrenal gland and observe which of the following?

A. It receives its arterial blood supply from the aorta only
B. Its central vein drains into the IVC
C. Its central vein drains into the left renal vein
D. It is in contact with the head of the pancreas
E. It lies external to the renal fascia

[26.2] After removal of a large portion of the stomach in a patient who has cancer, you are now examining the lymph nodes that receive lymph from the stomach. Which of the following structures receives lymph directly from the stomach?

A. Cisterna chili
B. Aorticorenal nodes
C. Celiac nodes
D. Superior mesenteric nodes
E. Inferior mesenteric nodes

[26.3] In a patient who has testicular cancer that has metastasized (spread) to the lymph nodes, which of the following would you expect to be involved first?

A. Lumbar (aortic) nodes
B. Aorticorenal nodes
C. Inferior mesenteric nodes
D. Common iliac nodes
E. Internal iliac nodes

Answers

[26.1] **B.** The central vein of the right suprarenal gland drains into the IVC, whereas that of the right gland drains into the left renal vein.

[26.2] **C.** Lymph nodes located along the several arteries that supply the stomach will have their lymph drain to the celiac nodes. Remember that the arteries that supply the stomach are all branches of the celiac artery.

[26.3] **A.** Tumor cells from either gonad that metastasize through the lymphatics will metastasize to the lumbar (aortic) lymph group. Remember the origin of the gonadal arteries is the abdominal aorta.

ANATOMY PEARLS

❖ The right suprarenal gland is closely related to the IVC, into which its vein will open.

❖ The left suprarenal vein drains into the left renal vein.

❖ Multiple arteries to the suprarenal glands arise from the inferior phrenic artery, aorta, and renal artery.

❖ Lymph from the gonads drains to upper lumbar nodes.

❖ Lymph above the pectinate line of the anal canal drains to the iliac nodes, whereas lymph below the pectinate line drains to inguinal nodes.

REFERENCES

Foster RS, Hunter JG, Spivak H, Smith CD. Open adrenalectomy. In: Wood WC, Skandalakis JE, eds. Anatomic Basis of Tumor Surgery. St. Louis, MO: Quality Medical Publishing, 1999:786–94.

Moore KL, Dalley AF. Clinically Oriented Anatomy, 5th ed. Baltimore, MD: Lippincott Williams & Wilkins, 2006:317–8, 341–3.

Netter FH. Atlas of Human Anatomy, 4th ed. Philadelphia, PA: Saunders, 2006; plates 266, 314, 317, 332.

A 27-year-old female notes a tender lump in her groin area that appeared approximately 3 weeks ago. She relates that she had a similar mass about 1 year ago that required minor surgery. On physical examination, she is afebrile, and inspection of the perineum shows a 3 × 2-cm fluctuant mass at the 5-o'clock position of the vestibule. It is mildly tender, red, and slightly warm to the touch.

◆ **What is the most likely diagnosis?**

◆ **What structures are causing the groin enlargement?**

ANSWERS TO CASE 27: GREATER VESTIBULAR (BARTHOLIN) GLAND ABSCESS

Summary: A 27-year-old female notes a tender lump in the groin that appeared 3 weeks ago. She had surgery for a similar mass a year ago. The patient is afebrile and has a 3 × 2-cm fluctuant, inflamed mass at the 5-o'clock position of the vestibule.

◆ **Most likely diagnosis:** Greater vestibular (Bartholin) gland abscess

◆ **Cause of groin lump:** Inguinal lymph nodes

CLINICAL CORRELATION

This young woman notes the appearance of an inflamed, perineal, or vulvar mass in the posterolateral region of the vestibule. She apparently had a similar lesion 1 year previously. These are very consistent with a greater vestibular (Bartholin) gland infection. The greater vestibular glands are located at the 5- and 7-o'clock positions of the vulva. If the ducts of the glands become obstructed, the glands may enlarge and become infected, usually with multiple organisms other than those responsible for sexually transmitted diseases. Lymphatic drainage of the vulva is first to the inguinal lymph nodes. Treatment for this patient is to create a fistulous tract to decrease the incidence of recurrence; the two most common methods are incision and drainage with a catheter left in place for several weeks and marsupialization of the cyst wall, which is suturing the inner lining of the cyst wall to the epithelium around the periphery of the cyst. Biopsy is typically not required in a young patient, but for vulvar masses or abnormalities in women older than 40 years it is required to rule out malignancy.

APPROACH TO THE VULVA

Objectives

1. Be able to define the boundaries of the perineum.
2. Be able to describe the urogenital triangle.
3. Be able to describe the lymphatic drainage of the perineum.

Definitions

Vulva: The region of the external genitalia of the female.
Greater vestibular glands: Bartholin glands; two small reddish bodies on the posterolateral aspects of the vestibule.
Marsupialization: Surgical procedure in which the inner lining of the cyst wall is sutured to the epithelium around the periphery of the cyst to promote cyst drainage.

DISCUSSION

The **perineum** is defined as the region of the trunk, between the thighs and buttocks, inferior to the pelvic diaphragm. It is bounded bilaterally by the **pubic symphysis** (anterior), **ischiopubic ramus** (anterolateral), **ischial tuberosity** (lateral), **sacrotuberous ligament** (posterolateral), and the **coccyx** (posterior). A line between the ischial tuberosities divides the perineum into **anterior and posterior urogenital** and **anal triangles**, respectively. Deep to the skin is the fatty layer of superficial fascia, a continuation of a similar layer in the abdomen (**Camper fascia**). In the abdomen, deep to the fatty layer is the membranous layer of superficial fascia (Scarpa fascia) that continues into the perineum where it is called **Colles fascia.** In the perinium, Colles fascia is attached laterally to the fascia lata of the thigh and to the posterior border of the perineal membrane and the perineal body. The perineal membrane is a thin but strong fascial sheet attached to the ischiopubic rami, thus stretching across the urogenital triangle. The potential space between the deep layer of the **superficial (Colles) fascia** and the perineal membrane is the superficial perineal pouch (space). Attached to the superior surface of the perineal membrane are the **deep transverse perineal and sphincter urethrae muscles** within the **deep perineal pouch** (space). The perineal body attaches to the posterior edge of the membrane at its midpoint (Figures 27-1 and 27-2).

Superficial to the perineal membrane, the **pudendum or vulva (external genitalia)** includes the **mons pubis** and **labia majora, labia minora, vaginal vestibule, bulbs of the vestibule, greater vestibular (Bartholin) glands, clitoris,** and the associated **ischiocavernosus and bulbospongiosus muscles.**

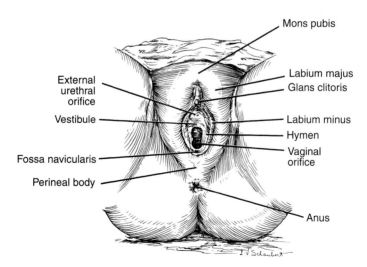

Figure 27-1. External female genitalia. (*Reproduced, with permission, from Decherney AH, Nathan L. Current Obstetric and Gynecologic Diagnosis and Treatment, 9th ed. New York: McGraw-Hill, 2003:17.*)

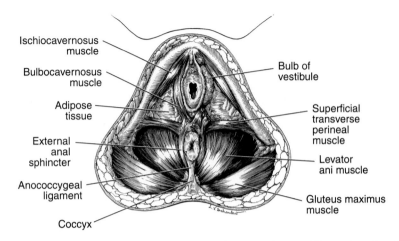

Ischiocavernosus
muscle

Bulbocavernosus
muscle

Adipose
tissue

External
anal
sphincter

Anococcygeal
ligament

Coccyx

Bulb of
vestibule

Superficial
transverse
perineal
muscle

Levator
ani muscle

Gluteus maximus
muscle

Figure 27-2. Interior view of female pelvic musculature. (*Reproduced, with permission, from Decherney AH, Nathan L. Current Obstetric and Gynecologic Diagnosis and Treatment, 9th ed. New York: McGraw-Hill, 2003:22.*)

The mons pubis is a rounded, hair-covered elevation anterior to the pubic symphysis formed by a mass of the fatty layer of the superficial fascia. Fat-filled posterior extensions of the mons form the hair-covered labia majora, which are united by anterior and posterior commissures. The space between the two labia is the **pudendal cleft.** Medial to each labia majora are the thin, fat-free, hairless **labia minora** that are filled with erectile tissue and surround the vestibule of the vagina, which contains the **urethral and vaginal orifices.** The labia minora are united posteriorly by **the frenulum of the labia minora or fourchette.** Anteriorly, the two labia minora are united by extensions that pass anterior and posterior to the glans of the clitoris as the prepuce and frenulum of the clitoris, respectively. The clitoris is composed **of paired cylinders of erectile tissue or corpora cavernosa attached to the ischiopubic rami as the two crura** and are surrounded by the ischiocavernosus muscles. The **corpora cavernosa** converge toward the pubic symphysis to form the body, which is sharply flexed inferiorly and terminates as the glans anterior to the urethral orifice. Superiorly (deep) to the labia majora and minora, at the margins of the vestibule, are the **paired bulbs of the vestibule.** At the posterior ends of the bulbs and partially embedded in them are the paired **greater vestibular (Bartholin) glands.** The bulbs and glands are covered by the bulbospongiosus muscles. A superficial transverse perineal muscle lies along the posterior edge of the perineal membrane and attaches laterally to the ischial tuberosity and medially to the perineal body. The components of the clitoris, bulb of the vestibule, greater vestibular gland, bulbospongiosus, and ischiocavernosus muscles are encased in the deep perineal or investing (Gallaudet) fascia. The bulbospongiosus, superficial and deep transverse perineal, and external anal sphincter muscles attach to the perineal body.

The **lymphatic drainage** of the perineum is primarily to the **superficial inguinal lymph nodes,** which lie inferior and parallel to the inguinal ligament. Efferent vessels from this group drain lymph to the **external iliac nodes,** but some lymph does drain to the **deep inguinal nodes,** which then drain to the external iliac nodes. Small amounts of lymph from deep perineal structures drain to the internal iliac nodes.

COMPREHENSION QUESTIONS

[27.1] A 34-year-old woman who has diabetes develops a "boil" on the right labia majora. Which of the following lymph nodes is most likely to be enlarged in response to the infection?

    A. Internal iliac
    B. External iliac
    C. Superficial inguinal
    D. Obturator

[27.2] Which of the following structures divides the perineum into the genitourinary and anal triangles?

    A. Levator ani muscles
    B. Superficial transverse perineal muscle
    C. Line from the ischial tuberosities
    D. Anal verge

[27.3] A 24-year-old woman is undergoing a vaginal delivery. A midline episiotomy is performed that incises into the perineal body. Which of the following muscles is most likely to be cut during this process?

    A. Superficial transverse perineal muscle
    B. Levator ani muscle
    C. Puborectalis muscle
    D. Pubococcygeus muscle

Answers

[27.1]   **C.** The primary drainage of the vulva is the superficial inguinal nodes.

[27.2]   **C.** A line between the two ischial tuberosities divides the perineum into the genitourinary triangle (anteriorly) and the anal triangle (posteriorly).

[27.3]   **A.** The muscles that attach to the perineal body are the bulbospongiosus, superficial and deep transverse perineal muscles, and the external anal sphincter.

ANATOMY PEARLS

 The clitoral structures, vestibular bulb, greater vestibular gland, and associated muscles are located in the superficial perineal pouch (space).

 The bulbospongiosus, ischiocavernosus, superficial, and deep transverse perineal and sphincter urethrae muscles are innervated by the pudendal nerve.

❖ The primary lymphatic drainage of the perineum is to the superficial inguinal lymph nodes.

REFERENCES

Moore KL, Dalley AF. Clinically Oriented Anatomy, 5th ed. Baltimore, MD: Lippincott Williams & Wilkins, 2006:433-41, 461–7.

Netter FH. Atlas of Human Anatomy, 4th ed. Philadelphia, PA: Saunders, 2006: plates 377, 379, 406.

Snell RS. Clinical Anatomy by Regions, 8th ed. Baltimore, MD: Lippincott Williams & Wilkins, 2008:400–2, 408–9.

A 20-year-old male reports that he has had a nontender, heavy sensation in his scrotal area for 2 months. He jogs several miles every day but denies lifting heavy objects. He does not recall trauma to the area, has no urinary complaints, does not smoke, and otherwise appears healthy. His blood pressure is 110/70 mm Hg, heart rate is 80 beats/min, and he is without fever. Heart and lungs examinations are normal. His back and abdomen are nontender, and no abdominal masses are detected. External genitalia examination reveals a 2-cm nontender mass in the right testicle that shows no light penetration with transillumination. The rectal examination is unremarkable.

◆ **What is the most likely diagnosis?**

ANSWER TO CASE 28: TESTICULAR CANCER

Summary: A 20-year-old male is noted to have a nontender heavy sensation in the scrotal area of 2 months' duration. He jogs several miles each day and denies lifting heavy objects, scrotal trauma, and urinary problems. A 2-cm, nontender, nontransilluminating mass is noted in the right testicle. The rectal examination is unremarkable.

◆ **Most likely diagnosis:** Testicular cancer

CLINICAL CORRELATION

Testicular carcinoma affects young men, usually between ages 15 and 40 years, and the presence of a painless scrotal mass is the most common presentation. A history of trivial scrotal trauma is not uncommon, which often brings the scrotal mass to the patient's attention. Testicular carcinoma should be ruled out before other conditions are considered, such as varicocele, spermatocele, hydrocele, epididymitis, or testicular torsion. Regular scrotal examination is advocated but rarely performed, and personal embarrassment often delays medical consultation.

APPROACH TO MALE GENITALIA

Objectives

1. Be able to describe the anatomy of the external male genitalia.
2. Be able to draw the blood supply and lymphatic drainage of the testicles.

Definitions

Transillumination: Passage of light through a specific tissue during examination with the object between the light source and the examiner.
Circumcision: Removal of all or part of the prepuce or foreskin.
Hydrocele: Collection of fluid in the tunica vaginalis of the testicle or along the spermatic cord.

DISCUSSION

The **male external genitalia** consist of the **penis** and the **scrotum,** which contains the **testes,** the male gonad. All of these structures lie within the boundaries of the **urogenital triangle** of the **perineum.** The relations of the **perineal fascia and spaces** (pouches) of the male perineum are similar to those described for the female perineum (see Case 27). For example, the membranous layer of the superficial fascia attaches to the posterior margin of the perineal membrane, the same three superficial perineal muscles are surrounded by the deep perineal fascia, and superficial and deep spaces are present. However in the male perineum, the fatty layer of the superficial fascia is virtually absent on the penis and is replaced by **smooth (dartos) muscles** in the scrotum. The membranous layer of the superficial fascia is continuous in the penis and scrotum as the dartos fascia (Figures 28-1 and 28-2).

The **penis** is **developmentally homologous** to the **clitoris** in the female and has many anatomical similarities. However, the **urethra traverses the corpus spongiosum.** The **penis consists of root, body, and glans**, which are formed from three cylindrical bodies of erectile tissue, each surrounded by a thick fibrous capsule called the **tunica albuginea.** Paired **corpora cavernosa** attach to the posterior portion of the ischiopubic rami (the crura of the penis) and converge anteriorly at the pubic symphysis. The paired bodies fuse with each other and are flexed inferiorly. The single **corpus spongiosum** begins as an expanded region called the bulb of the penis, which is attached to the inferior surface of the perineal membrane, and into which the urethra passes. The crura and bulb form the root of the penis. The corpus spongiosum with the urethra within it courses anteriorly to meet and fuse with the paired corpora cavernosa and form the body of the penis. The distal portion of the corpus spongiosum is expanded as the glans, which caps the distal ends of the paired corpora cavernosa. The external urethral orifice is at the tip of the glans. The **three fused erectile bodies are surrounded by a deep (Buck) fascia,** thin loose connective tissue and thin, somewhat pigmented skin. The glans is covered by a redundant fold of skin called the **prepuce (foreskin)** and is removed if a child is **circumcised.** The **posterior crural portion of the corpora cavernosa** are

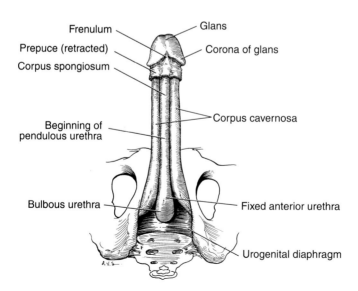

Figure 28-1. Ventral view of the penis. (*Reproduced, with permission, from Lindner HH. Clinical Anatomy. East Norwalk, CT: Appleton & Lange, 1989:498.*)

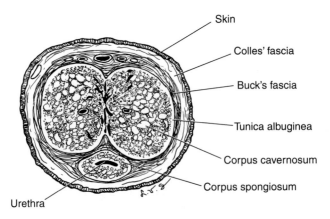

Figure 28-2. Transverse section of the penis. (*Reproduced, with permission, from Lindner HH. Clinical Anatomy. East Norwalk, CT:Appleton & Lange, 1989:500.*)

covered with ischiocavernosus muscles, and the **corpus spongiosum is covered by the paired bulbospongiosus muscles. Superficial transverse perineal muscles** are also present at the posterior margin of the perineal membrane and attach to the perineal body.

The **scrotum** is a sac of pigmented skin and the **dartos fascial layer,** which contains smooth muscle fibers that produce the characteristic wrinkling of the skin. The scrotum is posteroinferior to the penis and is divided into two compartments by an internal septum. Each compartment contains a **testis, epididymis, and the spermatic cord.** Each testis is ovoid with a thick fibrous capsule, the **tunica albuginea,** from which incomplete connective tissue septa divide the interior into lobules. The **lobules contain testosterone-producing interstitial cells (of Leydig)** and **coiled seminiferous tubules where spermatozoa (sperm) are produced.** The seminiferous tubules converge toward the posteriorly located mediastinum to form tubules (straight tubules, rete testes, and efferent tubules), which convey sperm to the **epididymis.** The **epididymis is the comma-shaped structure attached to the posterior surface of the testis** and is composed of the highly convoluted ductus epididymis. The testis and epididymis are surrounded by a closed, double-layered peritoneal sac embryologically derived from the **process vaginalis.** The inner portion or the visceral layer of the tunica vaginalis is applied to the surface of the testis and epididymis and is continuous posteriorly with an outer, parietal layer of the tunica vaginalis. A small cavity with lubricating fluid separates the two layers (Figure 28-3).

The epididymis is continuous inferiorly with the **ductus (vas) deferens,** which courses superiorly to enter the superficial inguinal ring. The ductus deferens in addition to the **testicular, deferential, and cremasteric arteries,**

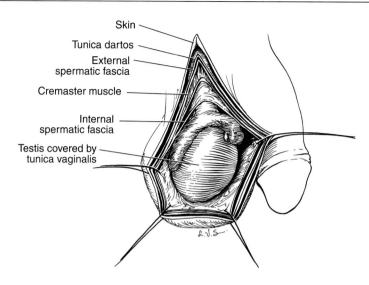

Skin
Tunica dartos
External spermatic fascia
Cremaster muscle
Internal spermatic fascia
Testis covered by tunica vaginalis

Figure 28-3. Layers of the scrotum. (*Reproduced, with permission, from Lindner HH. Clinical Anatomy. East Norwalk, CT: Appleton & Lange, 1989:501.*)

pampiniform plexus of veins, genital branch of the genitofemoral nerve, autonomic nerve fibers, and lymphatic vessels are components of the **spermatic cord.** The testis, epididymis, and spermatic cord are encased in three fascial layers derived from layers of the anterior abdominal wall (Table 28-1).

The testes are supplied by the **testicular arteries that arise from the abdominal aorta, just inferior to the renal arteries.** They course retroperitoneally to reach the deep inguinal ring, crossing anteriorly to the ureters and external iliac vessels. They traverse the inguinal canal to enter the scrotum through the **superficial inguinal ring.** Venous drainage of the testes is by the **pampiniform plexus of veins,** which follow a reverse course through the

Table 28-1
ORIGINS OF SPERMATIC CORD COVERINGS

FASCIA	ABDOMINAL LAYER OF ORIGIN
Internal spermatic fascia	Transversalis fascia
Cremasteric fascia and muscle	Internal abdominal oblique muscle
External spermatic fascia	External abdominal oblique muscle

inguinal rings and canal, to become paired testicular veins near their entrance into the abdomen. Eventually, a single testicular vein is formed that drains into the **IVC on the right side** but enters the **left renal vein on the left side.** Lymphatic vessels ascend along the paths of the testicular vessels, to drain lymph into **lumbar and preaortic lymph nodes** at the level of origin of the arteries. This high abdominal position of arterial origin and lymphatic drainage reflects the embryological site where the testes were formed.

COMPREHENSION QUESTIONS

[28.1] Which of the following is the male homologue of the female clitoris?

    A. Epididymis
    B. Vas deferens
    C. Penis
    D. Scrotum

[28.2] The scrotum appears to have a slightly pigmented and wrinkled appearance. What is the explanation for this appearance?

    A. Hyperkeratinized squamous epithelium
    B. The tunica albuginea
    C. The dartos fascia
    D. The pampiniform plexus

[28.3] An 18-year-old man is noted to have probable testicular cancer. He undergoes surgery. After incising the scrotum, the surgeon contemplates the approach to the parenchyma of the testes. Through which layer must the surgeon incise to reach the testicular parenchyma?

    A. Buck fascia
    B. Tunica albuginea
    C. Dartos fascia
    D. Scarpa fascia

Answers

[28.1]   **C.** The penis in the male is the homologue to the clitoris in the female.
[28.2]   **C.** The dartos fascia, which consists of smooth muscle, gives the scrotum its characteristic slightly pigmented and wrinkled appearance.
[28.3]   **B.** Each testis is surrounded by a thick capsule, the tunica albuginea.

ANATOMY PEARLS

 The root of the penis is defined as the crura and the bulb.

 The cremasteric muscle, which causes elevation of the testes in the cremasteric reflex, is innervated by the genital branch of the genitofemoral nerve.

 The testicular artery arises from the aorta just inferior to the renal arteries.

The right testicular vein drains into the IVC, whereas the left drains into the left renal vein.

REFERENCES

Moore KL, Dalley AF. Clinically Oriented Anatomy, 5th ed. Baltimore, MD: Lippincott Williams & Wilkins, 2006:451–61, 220–3, 227–30.

Netter FH. Atlas of Human Anatomy, 4th ed. Philadelphia, PA: Saunders, 2006: plates 380–2, 387.

Snell RS. Clinical Anatomy by Regions, 8th ed. Baltimore, MD: Lippincott Williams & Wilkins, 2008:402–8.

A 50-year-old female who has borne five children complains that she has noticed vaginal spotting of blood after intercourse for approximately the past 6 months. More recently, she has had a foul smelling vaginal discharge and indicates that her left leg seems larger than her right one. She previously had syphilis. She has smoked one pack of cigarettes per day for 20 years. Examination of her back shows left flank tenderness. The circumferences of her left thigh and calf are larger than those of the right. Pelvic examination shows normal female external genitalia and a 3-cm growth on the surface on the left lip of the uterine cervix.

◆ **What is the most likely diagnosis?**

◆ **What is the applied clinical anatomy for this condition?**

ANSWERS TO CASE 29: METASTATIC CERVICAL CANCER WITH URETER OBSTRUCTION

Summary: A 50-year-old female who has borne five children complains of a 6-month history of spotting after intercourse and foul-smelling vaginal discharge. She has had syphilis and is a smoker. Left costovertebral tenderness is present, and the left lower limb is swollen. Speculum examination of the uterine cervix shows a 3-cm growth of the left lip of the cervix.

◆ **Most likely diagnosis:** Metastatic cervical cancer

◆ **Applied anatomy for this condition:** Extension of the tumor to obstruct the left ureter and metastasis to iliac lymph nodes

CLINICAL CONSIDERATIONS

This patient's age, multiple pregnancies, and histories of smoking and a sexually transmitted disease are risk factors for cervical cancer. Vaginal spotting after intercourse is a common presenting sign for cervical cancer in a sexually active woman. Cervical cancer typically arises at the squamocolumnar epithelial junction, and the foul-smelling discharge suggests necrosis of a portion of this large tumor. Such a tumor can spread inferiorly to involve the vagina or laterally into the region of the transverse cervical (cardinal) ligament and can obstruct the ureter, which passes through the ligament. Further growth may reach the lateral pelvic wall. Involvement of iliac lymph nodes, in particular the external iliac nodes, may inhibit lymphatic drainage of the lower limb with resultant edema. Bilateral ureteral obstruction can lead to uremia, the most common cause of death in this disease. Radiotherapy is the primary treatment for advanced cervical cancer.

APPROACH TO INTERNAL FEMALE GENITAL SYSTEM

Objectives

1. Be able to describe the anatomy of the ovaries, uterine tubes, uterus, and upper vagina, including changes in their epithelial lining.
2. Be able to describe the anatomy of the lateral uterine support structures and related organs.
3. Be able to draw the lymphatic drainage of the uterus and upper vagina.

Definitions

Postcoital spotting: Vaginal bleeding after sexual intercourse, usually due to friable cervical tissue, and may be a sign of cervical inflammation or cancer.

Cervical dysplasia: Premalignant condition of the cervical epithelium usually induced by human papilloma virus, which over time, may evolve into cervical cancer.

Cervical cytology: Method of studying cells obtained by scrapings from the cervix.

Colposcopic examination: Method of visually examining the cervix with a binocular magnifying device, usually with the addition of acetic acid to locate areas of cervical dysplasia.

DISCUSSION

The **uterus** or womb is a thick-walled, hollow, **pear-shaped,** pelvic organ. Its main parts are the **body and cervix.** The **fundus** is the superior portion of the body between the openings of the uterine tubes, and the **isthmus** is the narrowed inferior portion of the body at its junction with the cervix. The narrow **uterine cervix** protrudes into the anterior wall of the upper vagina. The lumen of the cervix is the **cervical canal,** and its superior part opens into the uterine cavity as the internal os, and its inferior part opens into the vagina as the external os. The uterus is usually angled anteriorly in relation to the vagina, or **anteverted,** and the body and cervix of the uterus are flexed anteriorly with respect to each other, or **anteflexed.** This places the body of the uterus superior to the urinary bladder, often deforming it on cystograms. Posterior to the cervix is the rectum. The **vagina,** a tubular structure that is closed anteroposteriorly, begins at the **vestibule** and is directed posterosuperiorly to the level of the cervix. The protrusion of the cervix into the anterior wall of the vagina creates a circumferential gutter around the cervix, which, although a continuous space, is typically referred to as the **anterior, posterior, or lateral fornix.** The **urethra** is embedded in the **anterior wall of the vagina.** The columnar epithelium, which lines the uterine cavity and cervical canal, changes to a nonkeratinized stratified squamous epithelium at the margins of the external os. This type of epithelium covers the external surface of the cervix and lines the vagina (Figure 29-1).

The **uterine (fallopian) tubes** extend posterolaterally from the superolateral region of the uterus, the uterine horns. The uterine tubes are divided, from medial to lateral, into four regions: a **uterine or intramural portion** within the wall of the uterus, the narrowest portion or **isthmus,** the widest portion or **ampulla,** and the funnel-shaped **infundibulum.** The lumen of the infundibulum opens into the abdominal cavity, and its margin is arranged in a series of finger-like structures called **fimbriae,** one of which is usually attached to the ovary. The **female gonads, the ovaries,** lie close to the lateral pelvic wall, just inferior to the pelvic brim. Each almond-shaped ovary is supported by a **suspensory (infundibulopelvic) ligament,** which consists of the peritoneally covered ovarian vessels, an ovarian ligament, a derivative of the proximal portion of the embryonic gubernaculum, and the mesovarium portion of the broad ligament.

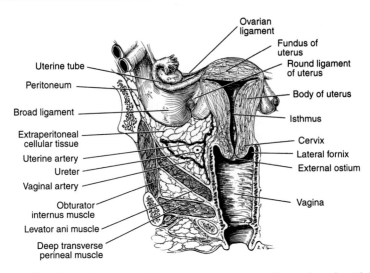

Figure 29-1. Frontal section of the uterus and vagina. (*Reproduced, with permission, from Lindner HH. Clinical Anatomy. East Norwalk, CT:Appleton & Lange, 1989:514.*)

The uterus, uterine tubes, and ovary are draped by a mesentery, the **broad ligament,** which passes from the sides of the uterus to the lateral pelvic wall to divide the pelvic cavity into anterior and posterior compartments. The broad ligament has three subdivisions: a shelf-like portion derived from the posterior layer of the broad ligament that attaches to the ovary, called the **mesovarium,** the portion of the broad ligament superior to the mesovarium that attaches to the uterine tube, called the **mesosalpinx,** and the portion from the uterus to the lateral pelvic wall, called the **mesometrium.** The continuation of peritoneum from the anterior surface of the uterus onto the anterior placed urinary bladder creates the **uterovesicular pouch.** Similarly, the continuation of peritoneum from the posterior uterine surface onto the anterior surface of the rectum creates the **rectouterine pouch** (of Douglas), the **most inferior recess of the abdominopelvic cavity in the female.**

The uterus and uterine tubes are covered with a layer of visceral peritoneum, but the ovary is not, being covered instead by a cuboidal germinal epithelium. The ovarian ligament is a cord-like structure between the layers of the mesovarium that extends from the uterine pole of the ovary to the uterine horn. Its continuation anteriorly to and through the deep inguinal ring and inguinal canal to the labia majora is the **round ligament of the uterus** (also derived from the gubernaculum). Beneath the peritoneum of the pelvic floor, paired condensations of connective tissue, the **uterosacral ligaments,** pass from the uterine cervix to the sacrum. An additional pair of condensation passes from the cervix to the lateral pelvic wall, the **transverse cervical (cardinal) ligaments.**

The transverse cervical ligaments lie in the base of the mesometrium, and the uterine vessels lie within or very close to these ligaments. The ureters coursing anteromedially on their way to the urinary bladder **pass inferiorly to the uterine vessels (mnemonic: water under the bridge)** and continue anteriorly, approximately 2 cm laterally to the uterine cervix.

The **blood supply to the uterus** consists primarily of the **paired uterine arteries** and the **ovarian arteries.** The uterine arteries arise from the internal iliac arteries and traverse through the transverse cervical (cardinal) ligaments. The fundus (top) of the uterus is supplied mainly by the ovarian arteries, which arise from the abdominal aorta. **Lymphatic drainage** from the fundus and body of the uterus is to the **lumbar abdominal nodes and to the external iliac nodes.** The **cervical lymph drainage** is primarily to **external iliac nodes,** but some lymph drains to **internal iliac and sacral nodes.** Drainage from the upper vagina is similar to that of the cervix, to the external and internal iliac lymph nodes.

COMPREHENSION QUESTIONS

[29.1] A 31-year-old woman is in her physician's office for a fitting for an intrauterine contraceptive device. The physician performs a pelvic examination to ensure that the device is placed in the correct direction. The physical examination shows that the uterine body is tipped toward the rectum and that the uterine fundus is tipped anteriorly. Which of the following describes the position of the uterus?

   A. Anteverted, anteflexed
   B. Anteverted, retroflexed
   C. Retroverted, anteflexed
   D. Retroverted, retroflexed

[29.2] A 45-year-old woman is having significant uterine bleeding from uterine fibroids. The radiologist performs an embolization procedure of the uterine arteries. Through which of the following structures do the uterine arteries traverse?

   A. Transverse cervical (cardinal) ligaments
   B. Uterosacral ligaments
   C. Vesicouterine fold
   D. Anterior vaginal fornix

[29.3] A 20-gauge spinal needle is placed through the vagina to assess whether there is blood in the peritoneal cavity. Which of the following describes the most dependent part of the peritoneum or pelvis?

   A. Vesicouterine fold
   B. Pararectal space
   C. Paravesical space
   D. Rectouterine pouch (of Douglas)

Answers

[29.1]   **C.** "Version" refers to the relation between the uterus and the vagina, whereas "flexion" denotes the relation between the body and the cervix. Thus, this uterus is retroverted and anteflexed.

[29.2]   **A.** The uterine arteries travel through the transverse cervical ligaments.

[29.3]   **D.** The most dependent region of the pelvis is the rectouterine pouch of Douglas. The procedure described is called a culdocentesis, in which the spinal needle is placed through the posterior vaginal fornix.

ANATOMY PEARLS

 The posterior vaginal fornix is in close relation to the rectouterine pouch (of Douglas), the most inferior portion of the abdominopelvic cavity in the female.

 The suspensory ligament of the ovary contains the ovarian vessels.

After passing inferiorly to the uterine vessels, the ureters course medially and lie approximately 2 cm laterally to the uterine cervix.

 Lymph from the uterine cervix and upper vagina drain primarily to the external iliac node group.

REFERENCES

Moore KL, Dalley AF. Clinically Oriented Anatomy, 5th ed. Baltimore, MD: Lippincott Williams & Wilkins, 2006:410–24.

Netter FH. Atlas of Human Anatomy, 4th ed. Philadelphia, PA: Saunders, 2006: plates 360, 362, 371.

Snell RS. Clinical Anatomy by Regions, 8th ed. Baltimore, MD: Lippincott Williams & Wilkins, 2008:364–7.

A 19-year-old female who has borne one healthy child is being seen at 7 weeks' gestation based on her last menstrual period and her complaints of vaginal spotting and lower abdominal pain. She denies the passage of any tissue through the vagina, trauma, or recent intercourse. Her medical history is significant for a pelvic infection approximately 3 years previously. On examination, her blood pressure is 90/60 mm Hg, heart rate is 110 beats/min, and temperature is within normal limits. The abdomen is normal, and bowel sounds are present and normal. On pelvic examination, the external genitalia and uterus palpate as normal. There is moderate right adnexal tenderness with palpation. Quantitative human β-corticotropin gonadotropin is 2300 mIU/mL, and transvaginal sonogram displays an empty uterus and some free fluid in the cul-de-sac.

◆ **What is the most likely diagnosis?**

◆ **What is the cause of the hypotension?**

ANSWERS TO CASE 30: ECTOPIC PREGNANCY

Summary: A 19-year-old female who has borne one child is seen at 7 weeks' gestation by last menstrual period and vaginal spotting. She has a history of a pelvic infection. Her blood pressure is 90/60 mm Hg, heart rate is 110 beats/min, and the abdomen is mildly tender. Pelvic examination shows a normal uterus and some moderate adnexal tenderness. Quantitative human β-corticotropin gonadotropin is 2300 mIU/mL, and transvaginal sonogram shows an empty uterus and some free fluid in the cul-de-sac.

◆ **Most likely diagnosis:** Ectopic pregnancy

◆ **Cause of the hypotension:** Ruptured ectopic pregnancy in the uterine tube with bleeding into the abdominal cavity

CLINICAL CORRELATION

An ectopic pregnancy results when a blastocyst implants outside the lumen of the uterus. The vast majority of ectopic pregnancies occurs in the uterine tube (95 to 97 percent), in the ampulla, the usual site of fertilization, or the isthmus, the narrowest portion. Any condition that might prevent or delay transport of the zygote to the uterus may cause an ectopic tubal pregnancy, and this patient's history of a pelvic infection (pelvic inflammatory disease) is a risk factor. Tubal ectopic pregnancies will usually rupture during the first 8 weeks of pregnancy, typically resulting in abortion of the embryo and intra-abdominal hemorrhage, with resultant hypotension and tachycardia. Tubal pregnancy in the narrow isthmus tends to rupture sooner than those in the ampulla and produce greater hemorrhage than implantation in the ampulla. Blastocysts implanted in the ampulla may be expelled into the abdominal cavity, where they may reimplant on the surface of the ovary, the peritoneum of the rectouterine pouch (of Douglas), mesentery, or organ surface. Severe hemorrhage typically results from an abdominal ectopic pregnancy, and the resulting hypotension may be emergent. The free fluid seen on ultrasound is blood that has resulted from the ruptured ectopic pregnancy.

APPROACH TO INTERNAL FEMALE GENITAL SYSTEM

Objectives

1. Be able to describe the anatomy of the uterine tubes.
2. Be able to draw the blood supply to the ovaries, uterine tubes, and uterus.

Definitions

Ectopic pregnancy: Pregnancy outside of the normal endometrial implantation site, usually involving the fallopian tubes.

Hemoperitoneum: Blood collecting inside the peritoneal cavity, usually leading to abdominal pain and irritation to the intestines.

Human chorionic gonadotropin: Glycoprotein molecule produced by the trophoblastic cells of the pregnancy.

DISCUSSION

The **uterine (fallopian) tubes** (see Case 29) extend posterolaterally from the uterine horns and are divided, from medial to lateral, into **four regions.** The **uterine or intramural portion lies within the wall of the uterus.** The **narrowest portion, or isthmus,** lies just laterally to the uterine horns. More laterally, **the widest and longest portion of the tube is the ampulla.** This is the **usual site of fertilization.** The most **lateral portion or infundibulum is funnel shaped.** The lumen of the infundibulum faces posteriorly into the abdominal cavity, inferior to which is the rectouterine pouch (of Douglas). The margin of the infundibulum is arranged in a series of finger-like structures called **fimbriae,** one of which is usually attached to the ovary. This attachment helps keep the infundibulum in close anatomical relation to the ovary, which in turn helps ensure that an ovulated egg will enter the lumen of the tube. The uterine tube is supported by the **mesosalpinx** portion of the broad ligament (Figure 30-1).

The ovaries, uterine tubes, and fundus of the uterus are supplied by the **ovarian arteries,** which arise from the abdominal aorta just inferior to the renal arteries (in a manner similar to the testicular arteries). The arteries descend, **crossing the ureters anteriorly,** and also cross the iliac vessels anteriorly at the pelvic brim. The ureters lie just medial at the pelvic brim. The arteries enter the lateral pole of each ovary, supply it, and continue medially between the layers of the mesosalpinx, close to its attachment to the uterine tube. It supplies the tube, continues on to supply the fundus of the uterus, and anastomoses with the artery from the opposite side. The **isthmus and uterine portions of the tube also receive blood from ascending branches of the uterine arteries,** which **anastomose with the ovarian artery.** This accounts for the increased hemorrhage with a ruptured tubal pregnancy of the isthmus. Venous drainage from these structures is primarily through the ovarian veins, which empty into the IVC on the right side and into the left renal vein on the left side.

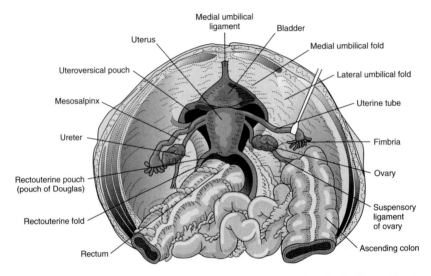

Figure 30-1. The female pelvis and internal organs (superior view). (*Reproduced, with permission, from Decherney AH, Nathan L. Current Obstetric and Gynecology Diagnosis and Treatment, 9th ed. New York: McGraw-Hill, 2003:33.*)

COMPREHENSION QUESTIONS

[30.1] A 22-year-old woman is noted during surgery to have a 3-cm ectopic pregnancy involving the ampulla of the fallopian tube. Which of the following best describes this location of the tube?

A. Portion within the muscle of the uterus
B. Portion that is narrowest and mobile
C. Portion that begins to widen distally and is the longest portion of the tube
D. Portion with finger-like projections

[30.2] Bilateral oophorectomy is performed in a woman who had ovarian cancer. To accomplish this procedure, the ovarian arteries were ligated. Which of the following describes the anatomy of the ovarian vessels?

A. Right ovarian artery arises from the right renal artery
B. Right ovarian vein drains into the vena cava
C. Left ovarian artery arises from the left internal iliac artery
D. Left ovarian vein drains into the vena cava

[30.3] A 3-cm ectopic pregnancy of the isthmus of the left tube is noted to
        have ruptured, leading to hemorrhage. The blood noted arises princi-
        pally from which of the following?

   A. Uterine artery
   B. Ovarian artery
   C. Uterine and ovarian arteries
   D. Neither the uterine nor the ovarian arteries

Answers

[30.1] **C.** The ampulla of the tube, which is the most common location of
        ectopic pregnancies, is the part of the tube that begins to widen at the
        distal end of the tube.

[30.2] **B.** Both ovarian arteries arise from the abdominal aorta. The right
        ovarian vein drains to the vena cava, whereas the left ovarian vein
        drains into the left renal vein.

[30.3] **C.** The uterine artery (ascending branch) and the ovarian artery anas-
        tomose to provide blood supply within the mesosalpinx to the tube.

ANATOMY PEARLS

The usual site of fertilization is the ampulla of the uterine tube.

The posteriorly facing ostium of the tube accounts for abdominal
ectopic pregnancies usually being in the rectouterine pouch.

The ovarian artery supplies the ovary, uterine tube, and fundus of the
uterus. Anastomosis with the uterine artery occurs in the region
of the isthmus.

REFERENCES

Moore KL, Dalley AF. Clinically Oriented Anatomy, 5th ed. Baltimore, MD:
    Lippincott Williams & Wilkins, 2006:424–7.
Netter FH. Atlas of Human Anatomy, 4th ed. Philadelphia, PA: Saunders, 2006:
    plates 360, 369, 371, 375.
Snell RS. Clinical Anatomy by Regions, 8th ed. Baltimore, MD: Lippincott
    Williams & Wilkins, 2008:363-4.

A 63-year-old male complains of a 6-month history of difficulty voiding and feeling as though he cannot empty his bladder completely. After voiding, he often feels as though he needs to urinate again. He denies urethral discharge or burning with urination. He has had mild hypertension and takes a thiazide diuretic. His only other medication has been ampicillin for two urinary tract infections during the previous year. On examination, his blood pressure is 130/84 mm Hg, pulse rate is 80 beats/min, and he is without fever (afebrile). The heart and lung examinations are normal, and the abdominal examination shows no masses.

◆ **What is the most likely diagnosis?**

◆ **What is the anatomical explanation for the patient's symptoms?**

ANSWERS TO CASE 31: BENIGN PROSTATIC HYPERPLASIA

Summary: A 63-year-old male who has hypertension complains of a 6-month difficulty in voiding and the sensation that he cannot empty his bladder completely. He has had two episodes of urinary tract infections but denies dysuria (burning with urination) or urethral discharge.

◆ **Most likely diagnosis:** Benign prostatic hyperplasia

◆ **Anatomical basis for the symptomatology:** Compression of the bladder neck or the prostatic urethra

CLINICAL CORRELATION

The **prostate gland** is the **largest of the male accessory sex glands,** and its secretions contribute to semen. This **encapsulated gland** is located in the pelvis, between the neck of the bladder and the sphincter urethrae muscle, and **surrounds the first part of the male urethra,** called the **prostatic urethra.** Enlargement of the prostate, benign prostatic hyperplasia (BPH), is a common condition in men older than 50 years and appears to depend on age and hormone level. A **prostate-specific antigen** blood test and a digital rectal examination (DRE) would be done to evaluate the gland's size and the presence of nodularity that might suggest carcinoma. Initial treatment after a confirmed diagnosis of BPH is often medical, with a medication such as a **5-α-reductase inhibitor,** which relaxes the smooth muscle within the stroma of the gland and thus increases urethral diameter. Other medications block the effects of testosterone metabolites on gland tissue, resulting in involution of gland tissue. In advanced cases, a surgical transurethral resection of the prostate may be required. Although no direct relation between BPH and prostate malignancy has been proved, both conditions occur in the same age group.

APPROACH TO MALE INTERNAL GENITALIA

Objectives

1. Be able to describe the anatomy of the internal male genital organs: ductus deferens, seminal vesicles, ejaculatory duct, prostate gland, and bulbourethral glands.
2. Be able to describe the anatomy of the male urethral tract.

Definitions

Prostatic hyperplasia: Benign enlargement of the prostate gland that, because of the capsule surrounding it, impinges on the urethra.

Urinary hesitancy: Abnormally long period required to initiate a stream of urine.

Transurethral resection of the prostate: Procedure in which the surgeon excises prostatic tissue from the prostatic urethra in an effort to relieve obstruction.

DISCUSSION

The **paired ductus deferenses traverse the inguinal canal** and enter the abdomen through the **deep inguinal rings,** where they retain a retroperitoneal position. They cross the external iliac vessels, superolateral surface of the bladder, and superiorly to the ureters entering the bladder (mnemonic: **water under the bridge**), and reach the posterior surface of the bladder, just anterior to the rectal vesicular pouch. The terminal portion of the ductus is dilated to form an **ampulla of the prostate.** Lateral to the two ampullae are the diagonally positioned, paired **seminal vesicles.** These accessory sex glands produce an **alkaline component** of semen, which neutralizes the usual acid environment in the vagina. The duct of each **seminal vesicle unites with the ductus deferens on each side to form the paired ejaculatory ducts,** which course anteroinferiorly through the prostate gland to open on the elevated seminal colliculus on the posterior wall of the prostatic urethra (Figure 31-1).

The **prostate gland is the largest of the accessory sex glands,** an inverted pyramid about the **size of a walnut.** The **base is located inferior to the neck of the bladder,** and the apex rests on the sphincter urethrae muscle. The prostate has a **thick fibrous capsule** surrounded by a fibrous sheath that is continuous with the puboprostatic ligaments. The levator ani muscle supports the gland inferolaterally, and the anterior surface is covered by fibers of the sphincter urethrae muscle. The prostate is anatomically divisible into **four lobes.** The **anterior lobe** lies anteriorly to the urethra and is a superior fibromuscular continuation of the sphincter urethrae muscle. The **posterior lobe** is midline, posterior to the urethra, and palpable by digital rectal exam (DRE). The **lateral lobes** on each side of the **posterior lobe** form the largest part of the gland and are also palpable by DRE. The **middle lobe is the wedge-shaped superior portion of gland between the urethra** and the obliquely oriented ejaculatory ducts and is **closely related to the neck of the bladder.** **Enlargement** of the **middle lobe** (as in BPH) causes pressure on the neck of the bladder. The multiple ducts of the prostate open onto the posterior wall of the prostatic urethra and comprise a major component of semen. The paired **bulbourethral glands** are pea-size glands embedded in the sphincter urethrae muscle, posterolateral to the membranous urethra. The ducts of each gland empty into the proximal part of the spongy (penile) urethra, in the bulb of the penis. **Their mucous secretions lubricate the urethra during erection.**

The **male urethra** is divided **into four parts.** The **preprostatic urethra** is a short continuation of the bladder neck. The **prostatic urethra,** the widest part, passes through the prostate gland, somewhat closer to its anterior surface.

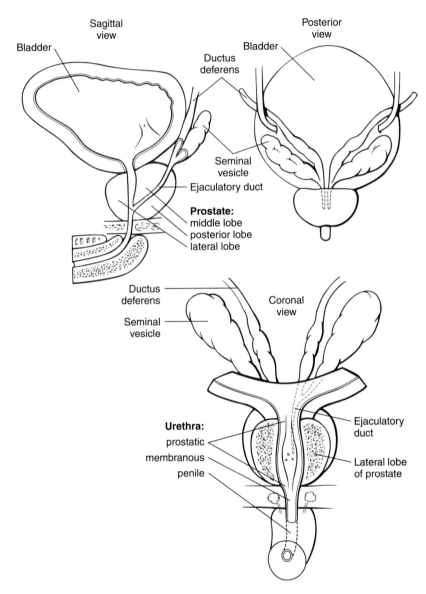

Figure 31-1. The prostate gland.

The posterior wall is elevated as a **fusiform ridge called the seminal colliculus,** on which are found the openings of the prostatic utricle (an embryonic remnant) and the paired ejaculatory ducts. The grooved portions of the urethra on each side of the colliculus are the prostatic sinus in which are found the openings of the prostate gland ducts. The third part is called the **membranous urethra** and is surrounded by the sphincter urethrae muscle or the external urethral (voluntary) sphincter. The fourth and longest part is the **spongy (penile) urethra,** which traverses the **corpus spongiosum** and terminates at the external urethral orifice on the tip of the glans penis. As the urethra enters the bulb of the penis, it widens to form the bulbar fossa into which open the ducts of the bulbourethral glands. The urethra widens again just proximal to the external orifice as the navicular fossa.

COMPREHENSION QUESTIONS

[31.1] A 66-year-old man complains of difficulty voiding and is noted to have probable BPH. Which of the following prostatic lobes is likely to be responsible for these symptoms?

A. Anterior lobe
B. Posterior lobe
C. Lateral lobe
D. Middle lobe

[31.2] A 48-year-old man is undergoing cystoscopic examination. As the cystoscope is placed into the urethra through the penile portion, which of the following tissues surrounds the urethra?

A. Prostate
B. Corpus spongiosum
C. Seminal colliculus
D. Sphincter urethrae muscles

[31.3] A police detective takes a scraping of some stains to be examined for alkaline phosphatase to assess whether these might be ejaculate. What is the source of alkaline phosphatase in the semen?

A. Prostatic gland
B. Bulbourethral glands
C. Seminal vesicles
D. Seminal colliculus apparatus

Answers

[31.1]   **D.** The middle lobe of the prostate is the part through which the urethra traverses and may be obstructed by BPH.

[31.2]   **B.** The longest portion of the urethra is the penile urethra, which traverses through the corpus spongiosum.

[31.3]   **C.** The seminal vesicles are the source of the alkaline phosphatase in the semen. The alkalinity helps to neutralize the acidity of the vagina.

ANATOMY PEARLS

❖ The posterior and lateral lobes of the prostate are palpable by DRE.
❖ The middle lobe may press on the bladder neck in BPH.
❖ The sphincter urethrae muscle extends superiorly to cover the anterior surface of the prostate.
❖ The bulbourethral glands lie adjacent to the membranous urethra, but their ducts open into the proximal spongy urethra.

REFERENCES

Moore KL, Dalley AF. Clinically Oriented Anatomy, 5th ed. Baltimore, MD: Lippincott Williams & Wilkins, 2006:405–9.

Netter FH. Atlas of Human Anatomy, 4th ed. Philadelphia, PA: Saunders, 2006: plates 361, 384–5.

Snell RS. Clinical Anatomy by Regions, 8th ed. Baltimore, MD: Lippincott Williams & Wilkins, 2008:352–6.

A 45-year-old female underwent surgical removal of the uterus (total hysterectomy) for symptomatic endometriosis 2 days previously. She complains of right back and flank tenderness. On examination, her temperature is 102°F, heart rate is 100 beats/min, and blood pressure is 130/90 mm Hg. The heart and lung examinations are normal. Her abdomen is slightly tender diffusely, but bowel sounds are normal. The surgical incision appears within normal limits. There is exquisite right costovertebral angle tenderness on palpation. Ultrasound of the kidneys shows marked dilation of the right renal collecting system and dilation of the right ureter.

◆ **What is the most likely diagnosis?**

◆ **What is the anatomical explanation for this condition?**

ANSWERS TO CASE 32: URETERAL INJURY AT SURGERY

Summary: A 45-year-old female who underwent total abdominal hysterectomy for symptomatic endometriosis 2 days previously has fever of 102°F and exquisite right flank tenderness at the costovertebral angle. The surgical incision appears normal.

◆ **Most likely diagnosis:** Injury to the right ureter

◆ **Anatomical explanation for this condition:** Probable ligation of the right ureter as it passes inferiorly to the uterine artery within the transverse cervical (cardinal) ligament of the uterus

CLINICAL CORRELATION

Approximately one-half the length of the ureter is located in the pelvis. It is at risk of injury at three pelvic sites during a hysterectomy. If the patient's ovaries are also removed (oophorectomy) at the time of the hysterectomy, the ureter is at risk where it crosses the common or external iliac vessels to enter the pelvis just medial to the ovarian vessels. The ureter is especially at risk deeper in the pelvis as it courses toward the urinary bladder inferior to the uterine vessels. Lateral extension of uterine pathology into the transverse cervical ligament increases the risk. The third site at which the ureter is at risk is as it passes laterally to the uterine cervix before its entrance into the urinary bladder. Hydronephrosis and/or hydroureter results from ureteral injury, and cystoscopic stent passage is often attempted first to relieve the obstruction, if possible.

APPROACH TO THE URETERS

Objectives

1. Be able to draw the abdominal and pelvic courses of the ureter.
2. Be able to describe the sites at which the ureter is anatomically narrowed and at risk during surgery.
3. Be able to describe the blood supply to the ureter.

Definitions

Hysterectomy: Surgical removal of the uterus.
Ureteral injury: Ligation, laceration, or denuding the ureter leading to ischemia. Ureteral obstruction can also occur from "kinking" of the ureter.
Intravenous pyelogram: Intravenous dye is injected and a series of radiographs are taken that incorporate the kidneys, ureter, and bladder. This procedure allows delineation of the anatomical structures and the function of the kidneys.

DISCUSSION

Each **ureter** is an inferior continuation of the renal pelvis, and the uretero-pelvic junction is at the inferior margin of the hilum of the kidney. One-half the total length of the ureter is abdominal, and the remaining half is located in the pelvis. The abdominal ureter descends **retroperitoneally** on the anterior surface of the **psoas muscle** and at about its midpoint is **crossed anteriorly by the gonadal arteries (testicular/ovarian).** The left ureter lies at the apex of the mesosigmoid. It enters the pelvis by crossing anterior to the external iliac artery (it may cross the common iliac bifurcation somewhat medially). In females, the ovarian vessels lie just lateral to the ureters as they enter the pelvis. After entering the pelvis, each ureter passes inferoposteriorly, anterior to the internal iliac vessels, to above the ischial spines. They then course anteromedially to the posterior bladder wall. In this course in a female, the **ureters pass inferior to the uterine vessels,** reaching the uterus from the lateral pelvic wall **(mnemonic: water under the bridge),** and lie approximately **1 cm lateral to the uterine cervix.** Externally, the ureters enter the bladder approximately 5 cm apart but course obliquely through the bladder wall such that their internal openings are but 2.5 cm apart (Figure 32-1).

Each ureter is anatomically narrowed in **three locations:** the **uteropelvic junction,** where the ureters cross the **external iliac vessels,** and as the ureters

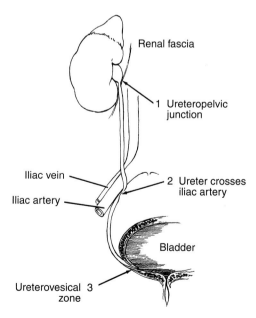

Figure 32-1. Course of the ureter. (*Reproduced, with permission, from Tanagh EA, McAninch JW, eds. Smith's General Urology, 12th ed. East Norwalk, CT: Appleton & Lange, 1988.*)

obliquely **traverse the bladder wall. Renal stones may lodge at these narrowed points.** The pelvic portion of the ureters is at surgical risk, especially in females during **hysterectomy** procedures. If an oophorectomy is performed with the hysterectomy, the ovarian vessels must be ligated, and **each ureter lies just medial to these vessels within the suspensory ligament of the ovary.** They may be inadvertently clamped, ligated, or divided at this site. The ureters are at risk as they pass inferiorly to the uterine vessels, in or adjacent to the **transverse cervical (cardinal) ligament,** where they may also be inadvertently clamped, ligated, or divided. The ureters are at risk in a vaginal hysterectomy as they course just laterally to the uterine cervix.

The arterial blood supply of the ureters is likely to come from any nearby artery, and its chief supply is derived from **ureteral branches from the renal, gonadal, aorta, common and internal iliac, and vesical and uterine arteries.** Ureteric branches reach the ureters from their medial side and divide into ascending and descending branches.

COMPREHENSION QUESTIONS

[32.1] A 39-year-old woman complains of hematuria and significant flank tenderness. She has a history of kidney stones. A CT scan depicts the abdominal portion of the ureter lying anterior to a muscle. Which of the following is most likely to be the name of this muscle?

A. Psoas
B. Serratus anterior muscle
C. Obturator muscle
D. Rectus muscle
E. External oblique muscle

[32.2] A dissection of the ureter is accomplished to excavate a large retroperitoneal mass. In isolating the ureter, the surgeon is attempting to ensure that the blood supply to the ureter is not disrupted. Which of the following best describes the arterial supply to the ureter?

A. Ureteral artery arising from the abdominal aorta
B. Ureteral artery arising form the external iliac artery
C. Ureteral artery arising from the internal iliac artery
D. No specific artery, but rather small branches from the nearby arteries

[32.3] A 30-year-old woman is noted to have an absent kidney. Which of the following findings is she also likely to have?

A. Absent unilateral ovary
B. Unicornuate uterus
C. Imperforate hymen
D. Inguinal hernia

Answers

[32.1]   **A.** The abdominal ureter lies anterior to the psoas muscle.

[32.2]   **D.** The ureter does not have any specific artery supplying it, but rather has small branches from the nearby arteries such as the renal, gonadal, aorta, common and internal iliac, and vesical and uterine arteries.

[32.3]   **B.** The urinary and paramesonephric ducts are in close proximity anatomically and relationally during embryologic development. Thus, a congenital abnormality in the kidney or ureter often is associated with an abnormality of the ipsilateral tube, uterine horn, or cervix. The distal vagina, vulva, and ovary are of different embryonic origin.

ANATOMY PEARLS

 The ureters are retroperitoneal along their entire length.

 The ureters are narrowed at three sites: ureteropelvic junction, crossing the external iliac artery, and as it is passing through the bladder wall.

 The ureters are at risk at three pelvic sites: where the ovarian vessels lie just lateral, passing inferiorly to the uterine vessels, and just lateral to the uterine cervix.

 Ureteral arterial branches reach the ureter from their medial side.

REFERENCES

Moore KL, Dalley AF. Clinically Oriented Anatomy, 5th ed. Baltimore, MD: Lippincott Williams & Wilkins, 2006:313, 391–4.

Netter FH. Atlas of Human Anatomy, 4th ed. Philadelphia, PA: Saunders, 2006: plates 340–1.

Snell RS. Clinical Anatomy by Regions, 8th ed. Baltimore, MD: Lippincott Williams & Wilkins, 2008:266–7, 347–8, 356.

A 54-year-old man complains of lower back pain that radiates down the back of his right leg. He states that the pain is worsened by coughing or lifting but relieved by lying down. He denies trauma to his back. On examination, the strength and sensation of his lower extremities are normal. During the examination, while the patient is lying on his back (supine), the patient complains of severe pain when his right leg is raised by the clinician.

◆ **What is the most likely diagnosis?**

◆ **What is the anatomical mechanism for this condition?**

ANSWERS TO CASE 33: PROLAPSED LUMBAR NUCLEUS PULPOSUS

Summary: A 54-year-old man has lower back pain that radiates down the back of his right leg, is exacerbated by intra-abdominal pressure (Valsalva), and is relieved by rest. He denies trauma. The neurological evaluation is normal, but his pain is elicited by raising a straightened right leg.

◆ **Most likely diagnosis:** Herniated lumbar disc (prolapsed lumbar nucleus pulposus)

◆ **Anatomical mechanism for this condition:** The ruptured intervertebral disc impinges on the nerve root as it exits from the vertebral canal.

CLINICAL CORRELATION

This patient experiences pain radiating down the back of his leg in the distribution served by the sciatic nerve. Hence, the syndrome is referred to as sciatica. The pain is caused by impingement of the nerve roots contributing to the sciatic nerve (L4 through S3). He has no history of trauma, and we do not have details of his occupation. Heavy lifting is often an associated factor. The pain is worsened by increased intra-abdominal pressure (Valsalva maneuver); thus, coughing and straining often exacerbate the symptoms. The straight leg raising maneuver elicits pain. Because this patient does not have neurological deficits, conservative therapy would include rest, physical therapy, and nonsteroidal anti-inflammatory agents. Most patients improve with this treatment. Lack of improvement, neurological deficits, or history of trauma or malignancy usually necessitates imaging of the spine. MRI is considered to be the most accurate means of examining this region.

APPROACH TO THE SPINE

Objectives

1. Be able to identify the features of a typical vertebra and the intervertebral joints.
2. Be able to label the components of the spinal nerve from spinal roots to primary rami.
3. Be able to locate sites where components of the spinal nerve can be compressed.
4. Be familiar with the dermatomes and the landmarks of the lower extremity.

Definitions

Supine versus prone: Supine is the position of lying on one's back, whereas prone is lying on one's stomach.

Herniate: To push through a containing membrane or tissue.

Sciatica: Syndrome caused by irritation to the roots (radiculopathy) of the sciatic nerve.

Symphysis: A secondary cartilaginous joint, in which two cartilaginous surfaces are held in place by a fibrous connective tissue, such as the intervertebral disc.

DISCUSSION

The **vertebral column** is a series of individual bones that are stacked vertically and held together by ligaments and muscles. There are 32 to 34 vertebrae (7 cervical, 12 thoracic, 5 lumbar, 5 sacral, and 3 to 5 coccygeal). The joints between each vertebra provide flexibility, but the vertebrae are held tightly in place by numerous supporting ligaments that provide strength and stability (Figure 33-1).

The **main features of a typical vertebra are the tubular body** and the **posterior arch** that surrounds and protects the spinal cord. The arch is composed of pedicles that arise from the **vertebral body and lamina that join at the midline.** Each vertebra has **seven processes:** three serve as attachment sites for muscles, and four serve as articular surfaces for adjacent vertebrae. The two **transverse processes** arise from the arch, where the pedicles and laminae meet. One spinous process emerges from the middle of the posterior arch.

Two types of joints support the articulation of adjacent vertebrae. The flat surfaces of the vertebral bodies join through a secondary cartilaginous joint, or symphysis. The bones themselves are separated by **the intervertebral disc,**

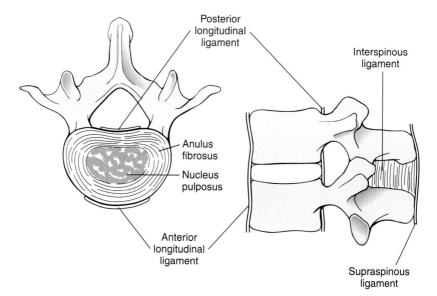

Figure 33-1. Major vertebral ligaments.

which has an **outer fibrous layer, the anulus fibrosus, that surrounds a soft inner layer, the nucleus pulposus.** The disc provides support for the joint but also provides flexibility and a cushion against the weight of the upper body. Secondary support is provided by the four articular processes. These processes also emerge from the posterior arch. Two are directed superiorly and two inferiorly. The superior and inferior processes of adjacent vertebrae join to form a zygapophyseal joint. This synovial joint provides strength with a limited amount of flexibility.

The pedicle and superior articular process together form a notch that is complemented by a second notch formed by the pedicle and inferior process. When two vertebrae are in apposition, the superior and inferior notches form the **intervertebral foramen.** This space is where spinal nerves emerge from the spinal cord to supply peripheral structures.

Peripheral nerve fibers arising from the spinal cord as **anterior (ventral) roots** are primarily **motor,** whereas the **posterior (dorsal) roots are primarily sensory.** These roots join to form the spinal nerve. In the cervical spine, the roots travel laterally to leave the vertebral column. The spinal nerve splits to form two mixed-function branches, a small posterior primary ramus and a larger anterior primary ramus. Nerves emerging from lower levels of spinal cord course inferiorly before they exit. This is because the **cord itself stops at about vertebral level L1.** Therefore the roots must travel nearly straight inferiorly before forming the spinal nerves of the lower lumbar, sacral, and coccygeal regions. As these numerous roots stream inferiorly, they form the **cauda equina.**

The symphysis between vertebral bodies is normally very strong because the intervertebral disc is reinforced by **anterior and posterior longitudinal ligaments.** However, in some people, these ligaments weaken, and the intervertebral disc pushes through. If so, the **roots** may be **compressed by the nucleus pulposus through the weakened anulus.** The most common result is stimulation of pain fibers in posterior roots. More serious cases may result in **paresthesia** (area of localized numbness), but rarely is motor function disrupted.

Although the actual site of injury is proximal, the brain perceives the information as coming from the region of the body innervated by the compressed root. Thus, with lumbar herniations, the distribution of this type of pain (radicular pain) tends to follow the **dermatomes of the lower extremity.** These areas progress on the anterior surface from **L1 in the inguinal region** to **L4 at the knee and medial leg** and to **L5 along the lateral leg.** On the posterior surface, **S1 is lateral on the thigh and leg, and S2 is medial. S3 through S5 are perianal.** Sensory fibers from a given spinal level spread into adjacent dermatomes. Therefore, in order to achieve complete numbness of a single dermatome, three adjacent spinal nerves must be anesthetized.

In this case, the patient experienced pain when, in the supine position, his straightened leg was raised. This sign indicates that slight mechanical stretching of the sciatic nerve is sufficient to enhance the effect of the herniated disc. Dorsiflexion of the foot exacerbates the pain. In some patients, straightening the contralateral leg may also cause pain in the affected leg, thus confirming radiculopathy.

Radiographic imaging can be used to confirm the herniation. Currently, the best modality is **MRI** because the herniation can be observed directly and MRI is a noninvasive procedure. With the widespread use of MRI, it has become clear that many herniated discs are asymptomatic. An older technique, myelography, is also used on occasion. This technique takes advantage of the fact that the dura mater covers the spinal roots and proximal spinal nerve. Injection of contrast medium into the cerebrospinal fluid (CSF) will infiltrate to the spinal nerves. Therefore, compressed nerve sheaths will not be filled by the dye, and the herniated disc can be observed indirectly.

COMPREHENSION QUESTIONS

[33.1] A 34-year-old woman is undergoing cystoscopic examination under spinal anesthesia. As the anesthesiologist places the needle into the subarachnoid space to inject the anesthetic agent, he goes through various layers. Which of the following describes the accurate sequence of layers from skin to subarachnoid space?

A. Skin, supraspinous ligament, interspinous ligament, posterior longitudinal ligament, dura mater, subarachnoid space
B. Skin, supraspinous ligament, interspinous ligament, dura mater, subarachnoid space
C. Skin, supraspinous ligament, intertransverse ligament, arachnoid space, subarachnoid space
D. Skin, interspinous ligament, anterior longitudinal ligament, dura mater, subarachnoid space

[33.2] A 45-year-old man complains of shooting pain down his right leg that worsens with sitting and coughing. He also has some numbness in the area. The physician tests sensation on the lateral thigh region. Which of the following nerve roots is being tested?

A. L1 and L2
B. L2 and L3
C. L4 and L5
D. S1 and S2
E. S3 and S4

[33.3] A 50-year-old man who has diabetes is having difficulty voiding urine. On examination, he has decreased sensation of the perineal region. Which of the following reflexes is the most likely to be affected?

A. Patellar tendon
B. Achilles tendon
C. Cremaster
D. Anal wink

Answers

[33.1] **B.** The sequence of structures is skin, supraspinous ligament, inter-
        spinous ligament, dura mater, and subarachnoid space.

[33.2] **C.** The lateral thigh is innervated by nerve root L5.

[33.3] **D.** The sensory fibers affected are from S2 through S4, which inner-
        vate the perineal region and supply the afferent limb of the anal wink
        reflex.

ANATOMY PEARLS

 The vertebral column consists of 34 vertebrae: 7 cervical, 12 thoracic, 5 lumbar, 5 sacral, and 3 to 5 coccygeal.

 Peripheral nerve fibers emerging from the spinal cord as anterior
(ventral) roots are primarily motor, whereas the posterior (dorsal)
roots are primarily sensory.

 The dermatomes of the lower extremities are L1 in the inguinal
region to L4 at the knee and medial leg and L5 along the lateral
leg. On the posterior surface, S1 is lateral on the thigh and leg,
and S2 is medial. S3 through S5 are perianal.

REFERENCES

Bickley LS, Szilagyi PG. Bates' Guide to the Physical Examination and History
   Taking, 8th ed. Philadelphia, PA: Lippincott Williams & Wilkins, 2003:594.
Moore KL, Dalley AF. Clinically Oriented Anatomy, 5th ed. Baltimore, MD:
   Lippincott Williams & Wilkins, 2006:478–553.
Netter FH. Atlas of Human Anatomy, 4th ed. Philadelphia, PA: Saunders/Elsevier,
   2006: plates 155, 162.
Snell RS. Clinical Anatomy by Regions, 8th ed. Baltimore, MD: Lippincott
   Williams & Wilkins, 2008:851–77.

A 68-year-old man complains of severe burning and stinging pain across the right side of his waist over a period of 2 days. Today, he notes a rash breaking out in the same area. On examination, there is a red rash with blisters starting on his back and curving down and across his right waist region.

◆ **What is the most likely diagnosis?**

◆ **What is the anatomical explanation for this condition?**

ANSWERS TO CASE 34: HERPES ZOSTER

Summary: A 68-year-old man has severe dysesthesia on his right waist for 2-day duration and, more recently, an erythematous vesicular (blister-like) rash.

◆ **Most likely diagnosis:** Herpes zoster

◆ **Anatomical explanation for this condition:** Reactivation of the varicella virus and infection of the skin following the dermatomal distribution, in this case, likely T11 or T12

CLINICAL CORRELATION

This 68-year-old man has clinical symptoms consistent with herpes zoster, also known as shingles. The chicken pox virus remains latent and may become reactivated years later due to illness, stress, or age. The varicella virus is reactivated from the dorsal root ganglia and initially causes a burning pain that follows the distribution of a dermatome, most commonly T3 through L3. Usually 2 to 3 days after the pain, a rash erupts that is erythematous and vesicular, and has a reddish blister-like appearance. Treatment of this condition may include corticosteroid therapy, which can help to decrease the inflammation and pain. Even after the skin lesions have healed, the patient can have significant pain, called postherpetic neuralgia. The pain can persist for months or even years. Treatment of postherpetic neuralgia is difficult, and therapies include topical lidocaine gel, capsaicin cream, anticonvulsant agents, or even nerve blocks.

APPROACH TO THE SPINAL NERVES

Objectives

1. Be able to draw the components of a spinal nerve.
2. Be able to draw the dermatomes of the thorax and abdomen.

Definitions

Dysesthesia: An abnormality of somatic sensation, for example, diminished sensation approaching numbness, an uncomfortable or painful response to a normal stimulus (as in this case), or a perceived sensation in the absence of stimulation.

Erythematous vesicular rash: Skin disorder characterized by redness and pustules.

DISCUSSION

Peripheral nerve fibers arise from the spinal cord as **anterior (ventral) roots,** which are primarily **motor,** and **posterior (dorsal) roots, which are primarily sensory.** These roots join to form the spinal nerve. The spinal nerve splits to form two mixed function branches, a **small posterior primary ramus and a larger anterior primary ramus.** In the abdomen, the posterior primary ramus innervates the intrinsic muscles of the back and the overlying skin. The anterior primary ramus projects anteriorly and inferiorly to innervate the muscles of the abdominal wall and the overlying skin (Figure 34-1). For a description of the peripheral distribution of spinal nerves, see Case 33.

After infecting the skin, the varicella virus is transported within the axons of sensory neurons back to the cell bodies, which are located in the **posterior root ganglia.** The virus periodically reactivates and is transported back out along the distribution of the spinal nerve that is carrying the sensory axons. Thus skin eruptions occur along the dermatomal distribution of the spinal nerve. In the thorax, the main dermatomal landmarks are the clavicle (L5) and nipple (T4). In the abdomen, the major dermatomal landmarks are the **xiphoid process of the sternum (T7), umbilicus (T10), and inguinal/suprapubic region (L1).**

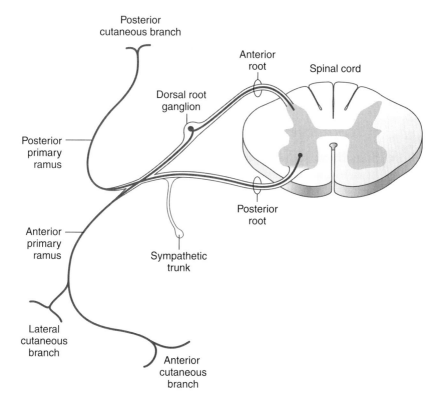

Figure 34-1. Components of a typical spinal nerve.

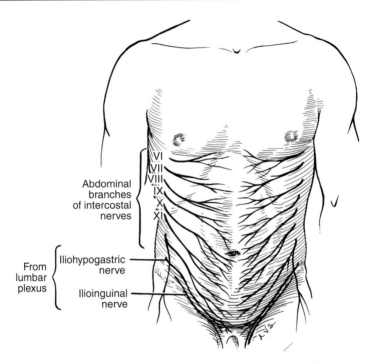

Figure 34-2. Distribution of cutaneous nerves over the abdomen. *(Reproduced, with permission, from Lindner HH. Clinical Anatomy. East Norwalk, CT: Appleton & Lange, 1989:302.)*

COMPREHENSION QUESTIONS

[34.1–34.4] Match the following nerve roots (A–F) to their locations on the body.

      A. C5
      B. C7
      C. T1
      D. T4
      E. T7
      F. T10

[34.1] Umbilicus

[34.2] Nipple

[34.3] Xiphoid process

[34.4] Clavicle

Answers

[34.1]   **F.** T10 innervates the skin around the umbilicus.

[34.2]   **D.** T4 innervates the nipple area.

[34.3]   **E.** T7 innervates the xiphoid process of the sternum.

[34.4]   **A.** C5 innervates the skin over the clavicle.

ANATOMY PEARLS

 Peripheral nerve fibers arise from the spinal cord. Anterior (ventral) roots are primarily motor, whereas posterior (dorsal) roots are primarily sensory.

 In the abdomen, the major dermatomal landmarks are the xiphoid process of the sternum (T7), umbilicus (T10), and inguinal and suprapubic regions (L1).

 In the thorax, the major dermatome landmarks are the clavicle (C5) and the nipple (T4).

REFERENCES

Moore KL, Dalley AF. Clinically Oriented Anatomy, 5th ed. Baltimore, MD: Lippincott Williams & Wilkins, 2006:206–10.

Netter FH. Atlas of Human Anatomy, 4th ed. Philadelphia, PA: Saunders/Elsevier, 2006, plates 164, 177.

Snell RS. Clinical Anatomy by Regions, 8th ed. Baltimore, MD: Lippincott Williams & Wilkins, 2008:21–8, 157–61.

A 7-year-old boy is brought into the emergency room for severe headache, nausea, and fever. His parent states that the patient had been in good health until 2 days previously. Bright lights seem to bother him. On examination, he appears lethargic and ill. His temperature is 102°F. Movement of the neck seems to cause some pain. The heart and lung examinations are normal. The patient refuses to flex his head so that his chin will touch his chest because the effort is too painful.

◆ **What is the most likely diagnosis?**

◆ **What is the most likely anatomical mechanism for this condition?**

ANSWERS TO CASE 35: MENINGITIS

Summary: A 7-year-old boy has a 2-day history of severe headache, nausea, fever, and photophobia. He appears lethargic and ill. His temperature is 102°F, and he has some nuchal rigidity.

◆ **Most likely diagnosis:** Meningitis

◆ **Most likely anatomical mechanism:** Migration of bacteria through the nasopharynx or through the choroid plexus

CLINICAL CORRELATION

This young child has a 2-day history of fever, headache, nausea, and photophobia. His general appearance is that of sepsis. The nuchal rigidity is suggestive of meningitis. These symptoms are caused by cerebral inflammation, ischemia, and edema. Increased intracranial pressure may cause lethargy and even seizures. The most common causative organisms are *Streptococcus pneumoniae* and *Neisseria meningitidis*. Previously, *Haemophilus influenzae* was the most commonly isolated organism, but, with the advent of the *H. influenzae* vaccine, this pathogen has been less of a factor. The diagnosis is made by lumbar puncture. Positive findings would be leukocytes (in particular neutrophils) isolated from the cerebrospinal fluid (CSF), and gram-positive organisms. A diffuse erythematous maculopapular rash that becomes petechial is suggestive of meningococcus. Rapid initiation of empiric antibiotic therapy is critical; the medication is aimed at the most common causative organisms and must penetrate through the blood-brain barrier.

APPROACH TO MENINGES AND CSF

Objectives

1. Be able to identify the meningeal layers.
2. Be able to draw the flow of CSF from the choroid plexus to the subarachnoid space.
3. Be able to identify sites where infection may spread into the cranial cavity.
4. Be able to describe the innervation of the meninges and the pathogenesis of headache.

Definitions

Ischemia: Decrease in blood flow to a tissue, generally due to blockage of the nutrient arteries.
Edema: Swelling due to accumulation of water in tissue.
Petechia: Tiny spots in the skin generally due to broken capillaries.

Choroid plexus: A tissue lining the ventricles of the brain that produces the CSF that fills the ventricles and the subarachnoid space.

Meningitis: A very serious infection involving the meninges, which may be caused by viruses or bacteria, and may lead to long-term consequences or death.

DISCUSSION

Within the cranial cavity, the **brain is protected by three meningeal layers.** The **dura mater, a thick fibrous membrane,** is the most **superficial.** Apposed to the deep surface of the dura mater is the **arachnoid mater,** which is a delicate thin membrane that is nearly transparent. The **pia mater** is the thinnest layer, and it is **directly apposed to the surface of the brain.** Three spaces relate to the three layers. The **epidural** space lies between the periosteum of the calvaria and the dura mater. Normally, the dura is closely apposed to the bone, so this is a potential space that can be expanded by blood or pus. Similarly, the arachnoid mater is closely apposed to the dura mater. The subdural space between the two layers is also a potential space. The **subarachnoid space** lies between the **arachnoid and pia mater.** This space is normally filled with CSF, which is the extracellular fluid of the central nervous system. CSF pooled in the subarachnoid space also serves a protective function by helping to insulate the brain and spinal cord from mechanical shocks.

CSF in the subarachnoid space is **produced** by the **choroid plexus,** in the ependyma of the lateral, third, and fourth ventricles. CSF produced in the lateral ventricles flows through the **interventricular foramina of Monro** into the **third ventricle.** The **cerebral aqueduct of Sylvius** then conducts CSF into the **fourth ventricle.** From there, fluid flows through the **foramina of Magendie and Luschka** into the subarachnoid space, where it surrounds the brain and spinal cord. The circulatory path ends at the arachnoid granulations, where CSF is resorbed back into the venous system. Most arachnoid granulations are found lining the large venous sinuses, but arachnoid villi may also be present at the roots of spinal nerves.

Meningitis is an **inflammation of the meninges,** but in practice the term refers to **infections of the pia and arachnoid layers,** usually involving the CSF (Figure 35-1). Infections reach the meninges by several routes. Most infections seem to be transferred through the vasculature (hematogenous transmission). On the arterial side, bacteria can infiltrate through the choroid plexus into the CSF. On the venous side, there are several routes from the face into the cranium. Normally, the veins drain superficially and inferiorly through the **pterygoid venous plexus** and **facial and retromandibular veins.** However, there are also anastomoses with the **superior and inferior ophthalmic veins.** These veins carry blood from the orbit into the cavernous sinus, which is in the anterior cranial fossa. Because veins in the face have no valves, some infections can reverse the normal flow of blood, so that **pathogens are carried into the cavernous sinus.** They can then infiltrate through the walls

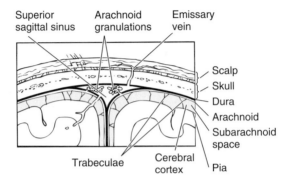

Figure 35-1. Cross-sectional view of meninges. (*Reproduced, with permission, from Waxman SG. Lange's Clinical Neuroanatomy, 25th Ed. New York: McGraw-Hill, 2003:158.*)

of the sinus into the CSF. A second route is through the nasopharynx. Mucosal infections can track through the **cribriform plate** into the anterior cranial fossa.

The **severe headaches associated with meningitis are due to increased intracranial pressure,** which **stretches the dura** and stimulates pain fibers from **cranial nerve V3** (mandibular branch of the trigeminal nerve) traveling with branches of **the middle meningeal artery.**

COMPREHENSION QUESTIONS

[35.1–35.4] Match the following anatomical spaces (A–D) to the descriptions of location.

    A. Epidural
    B. Subdural
    C. Subarachnoid
    D. Intra-arachnoid

[35.1] Between the dura and the calvaria

[35.2] Between the arachnoid and pia maters

[35.3] Between the dura and the arachnoid maters

[35.4] A 2-month-old baby is noted to have macrocephaly (large head) and developmental delay. On ultrasound, the baby has significant hydrocephalus. The pediatrician is suspicious of congenital stenosis of the aqueduct of Silvius. Which of the following are the most likely findings in this infant?

	RIGHT LATERAL VENTRICLE	LEFT LATERAL VENTRICLE	THIRD VENTRICLE	FOURTH VENTRICLE
A.	Dilated	Normal	Normal	Normal
B.	Dilated	Dilated	Normal	Normal
C.	Dilated	Dilated	Dilated	Normal
D.	Dilated	Dilated	Dilated	Dilated
E.	Normal	Normal	Dilated	Dilated
F.	Normal	Normal	Normal	Dilated

Answers

[35.1]   **A.** The epidural space is between the fibrous dura and the periosteum of the calvaria.

[35.2]   **C.** The subarachnoid space is between the arachnoid and the pia maters.

[35.3]   **B.** The subdural space is between the dura and the arachnoid maters.

[35.4]   **C.** The aqueduct of Silvius is between the third and fourth ventricles; thus, dilation of the lateral ventricles and the third ventricle is seen with aqueductal stenosis.

ANATOMY PEARLS

 The three meningeal layers that protect the brain are the dura mater (close to the skull), the arachnoid mater, and the pia mater (adherent to the brain).

 The epidural space is located between the fibrous dura mater and the periosteum of the calvaria, the subdural space is between the dura and pia maters, and the subarachnoid space is between the arachnoid and pia maters.

 CSF is produced by the choroid plexus, which is located in the lateral and fourth ventricles.

 The lateral ventricles connect to the third ventricle through the interventricular foramina of Monro. CSF flows through the cerebral aqueduct of Sylvius into the fourth ventricle and then flows through the foramina of Magendie and Luschka into the subarachnoid space.

 Meningitis is an infection of the pia and arachnoid layers, usually involving the CSF.

REFERENCES

Moore KL, Dalley AF. Clinically Oriented Anatomy, 5th ed. Baltimore, MD: Lippincott Williams & Wilkins, 2006:523–9, 923–7.

Netter FH. Atlas of Human Anatomy, 4th ed. Philadelphia, PA: Saunders/Elsevier, 2006: plates 99, 102, 104.

Snell RS. Clinical Anatomy by Regions, 8th ed. Baltimore, MD: Lippincott Williams & Wilkins, 2008:681–90, 752–3.

A 35-year-old woman complains of a 2-month history of hoarseness of her voice and some choking while drinking liquids. She denies viral illnesses. She underwent surgery for a cold nodule of the thyroid gland 9 weeks ago. Her only medication is acetaminophen with codeine.

◆ **What is the most likely diagnosis?**

◆ **What is the anatomical explanation for her symptoms?**

ANSWERS TO CASE 36: RECURRENT LARYNGEAL NERVE INJURY

Summary: A 35-year-old woman has a 2-month history of voice hoarseness and choking after undergoing surgery for a cold (nonfunctioning) thyroid nodule.

◆ **Most likely diagnosis:** Injury to the recurrent laryngeal nerve

◆ **Anatomical explanation for her symptoms:** Vocal cord paralysis

CLINICAL CORRELATION

This woman underwent surgery for a thyroid nodule. A cold nodule is defined as a mass that does not take up radioactive (i.e., "hot") iodine isotope. Surgery of the thyroid gland can sometimes injure the recurrent laryngeal nerve, which runs through the posterior superior suspensory ligament of the thyroid gland. The recurrent laryngeal nerve provides motor innervation to the larynx and sensory innervation to the laryngeal mucosa. A traction injury or inadvertent severing of the nerve leads to vocal cord paralysis. With injury to just one nerve, the vocal cord on the same side bows into a paramedian position instead of closing straight to the midline, leading to hoarseness of voice. When drinking, the patient may choke if the liquid is aspirated into the trachea. When vocal cord function does not return after 6 months to 1 year, then injection of the affected vocal cord with Teflon can be helpful.

There are four small parathyroid glands within the thyroid tissue, usually two in the left lobe and two in the right lobe of the thyroid gland. These tiny parathyroid glands secrete parathyroid hormone to maintain calcium balance. Inadvertent injury due to excision of the parathyroid glands can lead to hypocalcemia, manifested by fatigue, dyspnea (shortness of breath), brittle skin and nails, tetanic muscle contractions, seizures, or difficulty swallowing.

APPROACH TO THE NECK: THYROID GLAND

Objectives

1. Be able to identify the parts of the thyroid gland.
2. Be able to draw branches of the arteries and veins that supply the thyroid gland.
3. Be able to identify the main features of the larynx and list features that assist in respiration (phonation) or protect the laryngeal inlet during swallowing.
4. Be able to identify the course of the different branches of the vagus nerve (cranial nerve [CN] X) that innervate the larynx.
5. Be able to describe the consequences of injury to the recurrent laryngeal nerve and contrast with the consequences of injury to the superior laryngeal nerve.

Definitions

> **Cold nodule:** A region of the thyroid gland that does not take up hot iodine radioisotope (as visualized with thyroid scintigraphy) because the tissue does not contain follicular thyroid cells.
>
> **Ectopic:** Tissue that resides in an unexpected or abnormal location.
>
> **Aspirate:** To suck food or liquid into the bronchial tree of the lungs, possibly resulting in inflammation or pneumonia.

DISCUSSION

The **thyroid gland** is located at the **base of the neck.** It consists of **left and right lobes** connected by a **narrow isthmus.** During development, the **gland forms at the base of the tongue at the foramen cecum** and **descends into the neck** along the **thyroglossal duct,** reaching its final position **inferior to the cricoid cartilage** (vertebral levels C5 through T1). Occasionally, ectopic thyroid tissue will deposit along the duct. This sometimes manifests as a pyramidal lobe arising from the midline along the remnants of the duct.

As an endocrine gland, the thyroid receives a rich vascular supply. The **superior thyroid artery** is the **first anterior branch of the external carotid artery.** It descends laterally to the hyoid bone, giving off the **superior laryngeal artery,** which pierces the thyrohyoid membrane. The **superior thyroid artery** continues toward the gland lateral to the thyroid and cricoid cartilages. It crosses along the superior border of the thyroid and usually anastomoses with the contralateral superior thyroid artery. The **inferior thyroid artery** is a branch of the **thyrocervical trunk,** which arises from the first part of the subclavian artery. The artery ascends, giving off an ascending cervical artery, and then curves inferiorly to enter the thyroid gland from the posterior surface. There are many **anastomoses between branches of the superior and inferior thyroid arteries.** Rarely, an artery arising directly from the brachiocephalic trunk or the aortic arch, called the **thyroidea ima artery,** will ascend to supply the thyroid. The gland is drained by three pairs of veins. The superior and middle thyroid veins drain to the internal jugulars, and the inferior thyroid veins drain to the brachiocephalics.

The **thyroid lies anterior to the trachea (Figure 36-1),** a hollow tube that conducts air to the lungs. It forms from the inferior pharynx anterior to the esophagus. The wall of the trachea is supported by a series of cartilaginous rings. All of the unnamed rings have a **C shape,** leaving the posterior wall flexible to accommodate expansion of the esophagus during swallowing. Superior to the thyroid gland are the **cricoid and thyroid cartilages.** These are specialized structures that protect the underlying structures of the larynx.

The structures of the **larynx** serve two functions: to modulate expelled air to make sounds used in the **production of speech** and to **protect the airway** from food and drink passing to the esophagus. The **larynx** is formed from the **thyroid and cricoid cartilages,** and from several associated structures, including the **epiglottis** and the **arytenoid cartilages.** The **thyroid cartilage**

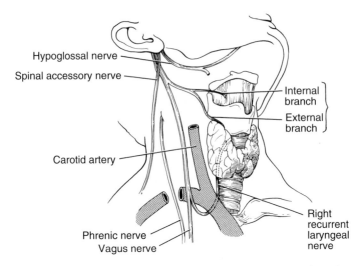

Figure 36-1. Nerves related to the thyroid gland. (*Reproduced, with permission, from Lindner HH. Clinical Anatomy. East Norwalk, CT: Appleton & Lange, 1989:138.*)

is the first and largest tracheal ring. It is a large C-shaped plate that forms the **laryngeal prominence** ("Adam's apple") anteriorly. **Inferior to the thyroid cartilage is the cricoid cartilage, which is the only tracheal ring that is closed posteriorly.** Posterior to the thyroid cartilage is the **epiglottis,** a cartilaginous structure that is bound to the thyroid cartilage by the thyroepiglottic ligament. The **arytenoid cartilages** rest on the superior margin of the cricoid cartilage and are held in place by capsules that surround the cricoarytenoid joint. The epiglottis attaches to the arytenoid cartilages through the quadrangular membrane. The free superior border forms the aryepiglottic fold, and the free inferior border forms the vestibular ligament (false vocal fold). The other major structure of the larynx is the **conus elasticus,** another broad ligament inferior to the quadrangular membrane. This ligament is the fusion of the lateral and median cricothyroid ligaments. The free superior border also attaches to the arytenoid cartilage and forms the **vocal ligament (true vocal fold).** The space between the two vocal folds is the **rima glottidis.** When the rima glottidis is wide (i.e., the folds are abducted), maximal air flow is permitted through the trachea. When the rima glottidis is closed (i.e., the folds are adducted), no air flows. When the **rima glottidis is narrow, the expelled air will vibrate the vocal folds and produce a sound.**

The intrinsic musculature of the larynx is for the most part devoted to fine control of the vocal folds to modulate pitch and intonation during speech. Perhaps the most important muscles are the **posterior cricoarytenoids,** which are the only muscles to abduct the vocal folds, and are **necessary to widen the rima glottidis for breathing.** All of the other muscles function to adduct the rima glottidis or modulate the tension of the vocal chords. The **lateral**

cricoarytenoids adduct the vocal folds. The transverse and oblique arytenoid muscles bring the two arytenoid cartilages together, which has an indirect action to close the posterior portion of the rima glottidis. The cricothyroids lengthen and tighten the vocal fold, whereas the thyroarytenoid relaxes it. The vocalis muscle runs under the vocal fold and produces local modulations in tightness (e.g., relaxing posteriorly while tightening anteriorly; Figure 36-2).

Several structures protect the trachea from food or liquid traveling to the esophagus. The first of these is the **epiglottis,** which deflects food laterally around the quadrangular membrane to the piriform recess and into the esophagus. The epiglottis itself is not sufficient to completely close off the laryngeal inlet. During swallowing, the **suprahyoid muscles** contract and, through the thyrohyoid membrane, lift the larynx up against the epiglottis. The **infrahyoid muscles** attached to the external face of the thyroid cartilage help to return the larynx to its resting position.

Most of these intrinsic laryngeal muscles are innervated by the **recurrent laryngeal nerve,** a branch of the **vagus nerve (CN X).** The only exception is the cricothyroid, which is innervated by the external branch of the superior laryngeal nerve, also a branch of the vagus. Thus, **damage to the superior laryngeal nerve** will affect the quality of the voice, particularly the ability to reach high tones. More significantly, damage to the **recurrent laryngeal nerve will impair** the ability to abduct the vocal folds, possibly leading to respiratory distress if the injury is bilateral. Unilateral damage to the recurrent laryngeal will result in inability to tightly adduct the two vocal folds, resulting

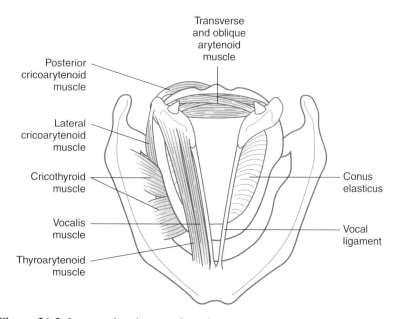

Figure 36-2. Larynx showing vocal cords.

in **hoarseness.** In addition, the **protective function of the rima glottidis may be lost,** and food or liquid that does not go down the esophagus may flow into the trachea and cause a **choking response.** In extreme cases, **aspiration pneumonia** may result.

Sensory innervation of the larynx is also mediated by the vagus nerve. In the **supraglottic region** (above the vocal fold), the mucosa is innervated by the internal branch of the superior laryngeal nerve. In the **infraglottic region** (below the fold), the mucosa is innervated by the **recurrent laryngeal nerve.** Thus, damage to the superior and recurrent laryngeal nerves may also have deficits in reflex behaviors that depend on sensory input from the larynx.

COMPREHENSION QUESTIONS

[36.1] Which of the following muscles is most important to allow air movement through the larynx?

   A. Posterior cricoarytenoids
   B. Lateral cricoarytenoids
   C. Cricothyroid muscle
   D. Infrahyoid muscles

[36.2] A 33-year-old woman underwent partial thyroidectomy for hyperthyroidism in which the thyroid failed to take up radioactive iodine. She is noted to have some hoarseness of voice 1 month later. Which of the following is the most likely explanation?

   A. Endotracheal tube trauma to the vocal cords
   B. Injury to the cricoid cartilage
   C. Injury to the thyroid cartilage
   D. Injury to the recurrent laryngeal nerve

[36.3] A 15-year-old boy is eating a fish dinner and inadvertently has a bone "caught in his throat." He complains of significant pain above the vocal cords. Which of the following nerves is responsible for carrying the sensation for this pain?

   A. Superior laryngeal nerve
   B. Recurrent laryngeal nerve
   C. Spinal accessory nerve
   D. Hypoglossal nerve

[36.4] A 25-year-old woman underwent surgery for a thyroid nodule. Two months later, she complains of dryness of skin and muscle spasms. Which of the following is the most likely explanation?

   A. Low serum magnesium
   B. Low serum calcium
   C. Low serum potassium
   D. Low serum sodium
   E. Low serum glucose

Answers

[36.1]   **A.** The posterior cricoarytenoid muscles are the only muscles that abduct the vocal folds and are necessary to widen the rima glottidis for breathing.

[36.2]   **D.** Injury to the recurrent laryngeal nerve is common during thyroid surgery and may lead to the inability to tightly adduct the two vocal folds, resulting in hoarseness. In addition, the protective function of the rima glottidis may be lost, and food or liquid that does not go down the esophagus may flow into the trachea and cause a choking response.

[36.3]   **A.** The laryngeal mucosa above the vocal cords is innervated by the superior laryngeal nerve, whereas mucosa below the vocal cords is innervated by the recurrent laryngeal nerve.

[36.4]   **B.** This patient likely has hypocalcemia due to excision of the parathyroid glands.

ANATOMY PEARLS

❖   The right recurrent nerve is located more laterally than the left recurrent nerve because of the course of the right subclavian artery.

❖   The posterior cricoarytenoids are the only muscles to abduct the vocal folds and are necessary to widen the rima glottidis for breathing.

❖   Most of the intrinsic laryngeal muscles are innervated by the recurrent laryngeal nerve, a branch of the vagus nerve (CN X).

❖   Bilateral injury to the recurrent laryngeal nerves may lead to respiratory distress, whereas unilateral injury results in hoarseness.

❖   Injury to the recurrent laryngeal nerve may affect the protective function of the rima glottidis, increasing the opportunity for a choking response.

REFERENCES

Moore KL, Dalley AF. Clinically Oriented Anatomy, 5th ed. Baltimore, MD: Lippincott Williams & Wilkins, 2006:1076–89.

Netter FH. Atlas of Human Anatomy, 4th ed. Philadelphia, PA: Saunders/Elsevier, 2006:plates 75–77.

Snell RS. Clinical Anatomy by Regions, 8th ed. Baltimore, MD: Lippincott Williams & Wilkins, 2008:802–9, 817–21.

A 59-year-old man complains of numbness of his right arm and slurred speech for a 4-hour duration. On examination, he has a blood pressure of 150/90 mm Hg and a normal body temperature. His heart has a regular rate and rhythm. Auscultation of the neck reveals a blowing sound bilaterally.

◆ **What is the most likely diagnosis?**

◆ **What is the most likely anatomical mechanism for this condition?**

ANSWERS TO CASE 37: CAROTID INSUFFICIENCY

Summary: A 59-year-old man who has hypertension complains of numbness of his right arm and slurred speech for a 4-hour duration. He has carotid bruits bilaterally.

◆ **Most likely diagnosis:** Transient ischemic attack

◆ **Most likely anatomical mechanism:** Left carotid insufficiency leading to ischemia of the left cerebral hemisphere

CLINICAL CORRELATION

This 59-year-old man has a 4-hour history of right arm numbness and slurred speech. This suggests ischemia of the left cerebral hemisphere including the speech area. If the deficits were to resolve before 24 hours, it would be called a transient ischemic attack. If the deficits were to continue beyond 24 hours, it would be called a cerebrovascular accident, or stroke. The two major types of strokes are ischemic and hemorrhagic. Differentiating between the two is important because fibrinolytic therapy (medication that dissolves blood clots) would be contraindicated with hemorrhagic strokes. Ischemic strokes can be caused by atherosclerosis or emboli. In this patient, the bruits identified on the carotid arteries are likely due to increased rate and turbulence of blood flow through the stenotic vessels. Immediate management of this patient would include administration of an antiplatelet medication such as aspirin and/or clopidogrel. An emergency computer tomographic (CT) scan of the head can help to differentiate between ischemic and hemorrhagic stroke, and fibrinolytic therapy can be considered if a cerebral hemorrhage is not found. After stabilization of the patient, carotid endarterectomy surgery may be indicated.

APPROACH TO THE NECK: VASCULATURE

Objectives

1. Be able to review the somatotopic organization of sensory and motor regions in the brain.
2. Be able to list the branches of the common carotid artery and the vascular supply to the brain and identify the sites most susceptible to formation of atherosclerotic plaques.
3. Be able to describe structures in the anterior triangle of the neck that relate to the carotid artery and sheath.

Definitions

Auscultation: Procedure of listening to the body during the physical examination, generally through a stethoscope.

Bruits: An abnormal sound heard through the stethoscope, generally a "whoosh."

Somatotopic: An orderly mapping of the body surface onto an internal organ, usually a region of the brain.

Ansa cervicalis: A loop formed superficially in the carotid sheath by branches of cervical spinal nerves innervating the strap muscles.

DISCUSSION

The major structural features of the **brain** include the **cerebrum and cerebellum.** The cerebrum is involved in the major functions of **sensory perception, motor control,** and the associational processing that integrates the two. The cerebellum is primarily involved in **motor control.** The surface or cortex of the cerebrum is folded into a number of ridges (**gyri**) separated by valleys (**sulci**) of different depths. The brain is divided into **lobes** named for the overlying cranial bones: **frontal, temporal, parietal, and occipital.** The central sulcus separates the frontal from the parietal lobes. The **precentral gyrus** controls **voluntary motion,** whereas the **postcentral gyrus is the site of somatosensory perception.**

The sensory and motor areas are arranged according to a somatotopic organization. The **lower extremity** is represented **medially along the gyrus,** the **upper extremity more laterally,** and the **head and neck are represented most laterally.** The **tracts** going to and from the sensory and motor areas **cross in the lower brain and spinal cord to control the opposite side of the body.** Another important region is the **motor speech area (Broca area),** which is a **small gyrus in the anterior parietal cortex of the left brain,** called the **operculum,** just superior to the temporal lobe. These basic organizational features are important because they help physicians to identify the region of the brain damaged by a stroke or hemorrhage. Thus, numbness or paralysis of the right upper extremity indicates damage on the left side of the brain. Damage on the left side of the brain will frequently involve the motor speech area.

The **blood supply to the brain** is from the **common carotid and the vertebral arteries** (Figure 37-1). The two ascend separately through the neck. The **vertebral artery** ascends through the **transverse foramina of the cervical vertebrae** without giving off any major branches. It then curves medially to ascend through the foramen magnum. The paired **vertebral arteries fuse to form the basilar artery.** The common carotid bifurcates at about the level of the hyoid bone (vertebrae C3 and C4). The external carotid ascends to provide branches to structures outside the cranium. The **internal carotid** ascends without major branches to enter the cranium through the carotid canal. After a relatively tortuous course through the sphenoid bone and the cavernous sinus, the

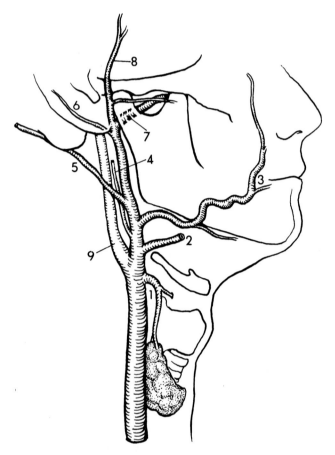

Figure 37-1. Branches of the external carotid artery: 1 = superior thyroid, 2 = lingual, 3 = facial, 4 = ascending pharyngeal, 5 = occipital, 6 = posterior auricular, 7 = maxillary, 8 = superficial temporal, 9 = internal carotid. (*Reproduced, with permission, from the University of Texas Health Science Center, Houston Medical School.*)

internal carotid emerges into the **middle cranial fossa.** In the region of the sella turcica and surrounding the pituitary stalk, the **vertebral and carotid circulations anastomose through a complex structure called the circle of Willis.** The circle of Willis is formed posteriorly by the bifurcation of the basilar into left and right posterior cerebral arteries. It forms anteriorly with the internal carotids, which bifurcate into the anterior and middle cerebral arteries. The left and right anterior cerebrals anastomose through the anterior communicating branch. The middle cerebral and posterior cerebral arteries anastomose through the posterior communicating branch.

The carotids are susceptible to occlusion as a result of atherosclerotic disease. The most common sites of occlusion are the bifurcation of the internal and external carotids and the bifurcation of the anterior and middle cerebral arteries. Occasionally, small pieces of an atherosclerotic plaque will break off (**emboli**) and obstruct a smaller artery. The **middle cerebral artery and its branches are most commonly** affected by this process. This artery ascends through the Sylvian fissure along the superior border of the temporal lobe. A major branch runs lateral to medial in the central sulcus. As a consequence, many strokes produce deficits in movement and sensation of the face and upper extremities and in language. More severe damage may also affect the lower extremity.

The carotid arteries are palpated in the anterior triangle of the neck. The **sternocleidomastoid muscle (SCM) separates the superficial neck into anterior and posterior triangles. The anterior triangle is further divided by the omohyoid and digastric muscles into four additional triangles: submental, submandibular, muscular, and carotid.** The common carotid artery ascends in the neck deep to the contents of the muscular triangle. These muscles are the sternothyroid, sternohyoid, and superior belly of omohyoid. It then goes through the carotid triangle, which is bordered by the superior belly of omohyoid, posterior belly of digastric, and sternocleidomastoid.

The **common carotid bifurcates** at the **level of the hyoid bone (C3),** and the internal carotid continues posteriorly. The carotids are contained within the **carotid sheath.** This fascial membrane forms from the other three layers of deep fascia that are in the neck: superficial layer of deep fascia, prevertebral fascia, and pretracheal/buccopharyngeal fascia. Also contained in the carotid sheath are the internal jugular vein and the vagus nerve (CN X). The vein is larger than the artery and lies more superficially. Several other cranial nerves have a structural relation to the carotid sheath. These include the glossopharyngeal (CN IX) and spinal accessory (CN XI) nerves, which exit with the vagus through the jugular foramen. The sinus branch of the glossopharyngeal nerve courses within the sheath to innervate the carotid body and sinus. The hypoglossal nerve (CN XII) passes deep to the carotid sheath as it projects anteriorly into the submandibular triangle. The sympathetic trunk lies deep to the carotid sheath on the surface of the prevertebral muscles. The superior and inferior roots of the ansa cervicalis, from spinal nerves C2 to C4, typically form the loop within the anterior surface of the carotid sheath before giving off branches to the infrahyoid muscles.

COMPREHENSION QUESTIONS

[37.1] A 47-year-old man complains of right arm weakness and difficulty speaking (expressive aphasia). Which of the following arteries is most likely affected?

    A. Vertebral
    B. Posterior cerebral
    C. Middle cerebral
    D. Anterior cerebral

[37.2] A surgeon is performing a carotid endarterectomy in a 55-year-old man who has carotid artery occlusion. In approaching the internal carotid artery, the surgeon severs a nerve embedded in the carotid sheath. Which nerve was severed?

    A. Superior laryngeal
    B. Vagus
    C. Sympathetic trunk
    D. Ansa cervicalis
    E. Recurrent laryngeal

[37.3] A 44-year-old man falls from a tree and develops a severe scalp hematoma. The superficial temporal artery continues to bleed internally because the man takes warfarin sodium (Coumadin) for an artificial heart valve. Which of the following arteries may be ligated to control the bleeding?

    A. Internal carotid
    B. External carotid
    C. Occipital
    D. Maxillary

Answers

[37.1] **C.** The middle cerebral artery supplies the temporal and parietal regions that contain Broca area (the speech center).

[37.2] **D.** The ansa cervicalis is a branch of the cervical plexus that innervates the infrahyoid strap muscles. The superior root generally descends within the carotid sheath superficially to the internal jugular vein. Therefore, this nerve is at risk during surgical approaches to the internal carotid artery.

[37.3] **B.** The external carotid artery divides into two branches: the maxillary artery and the superficial temporal artery.

REFERENCES

Moore KL, Dalley AF. Clinically Oriented Anatomy, 5th ed. Baltimore, MD: Lippincott Williams & Wilkins, 2006:927–32, 1067–72.

Netter FH. Atlas of Human Anatomy, 4th ed. Philadelphia, PA: Saunders/Elsevier, 2006:plates 105, 136, 142.

Snell RS. Clinical Anatomy by Regions, 8th ed. Baltimore, MD: Lippincott Williams & Wilkins, 2008:750–1.

A 3-month-old girl is noted by the pediatrician to have a stiff neck for a 2-month duration. The mother states that the neck seems to be pulled to the right. On examination, the baby's right ear is tilted toward her right side, but the baby's face is turned toward the left. Palpation of the neck reveals a nontender mass of the right anterior neck region.

◆ **What is the most likely diagnosis?**

◆ **What is the anatomical structure affected?**

ANSWERS TO CASE 38: TORTICOLLIS

Summary: A 3-month-old girl's head seems to be flexed to the right and her head rotated to the left. Palpation of the neck reveals a nontender mass of the right anterior neck region.

◆ **Most likely diagnosis:** Torticollis

◆ **Anatomical structure affected:** Sternocleidomastoid muscle (SCM)

CLINICAL CORRELATION

Torticollis is a deformity usually observed in children as lateral flexion and rotation of the head and neck. Congenital torticollis has an incidence of 3 to 5 per 1000 births. It is thought to be due to a fibrosis of the SCM that develops during infancy and causes shortening of the muscle. A mass can be palpated (about the size of an olive) about 66 percent of the time at the SCM. The etiology is unclear, although it may be associated with breech babies or difficult deliveries. The result is that the baby's head is flexed laterally toward the affected side and rotated contralaterally. Facial asymmetry may be noted. Physical therapy can help in most cases, but surgery is needed in rare cases.

APPROACH TO THE TRIANGLE NECK: ANTERIOR

Objectives

1. Be able to identify surface landmarks of the anterior neck.
2. Be able to describe the actions of the SCM.

Definitions

Fibrosis: Abnormal growth of fibrous connective tissue in response to trauma or infection.

Anterior neck: Portion of the neck anterior to the trapezius muscle. Within the anterior neck are two triangles, the anterior triangle contains structures anterior to the SCM, and the posterior triangle contains structures posterior to the SCM.

DISCUSSION

An important surface landmark on the anterior surface of the neck is the **SCM,** which divides the anterior neck into **anterior and posterior triangles.** The superior head of the muscle attaches to the mastoid process of the temporal bone. Inferiorly, the muscle splits to attach separately to the manubrium of the sternum and the clavicle (Figure 38-1).

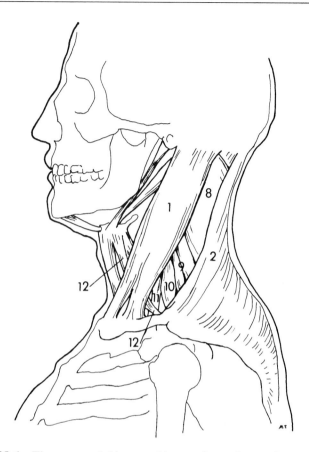

Figure 38-1. The sternocleidomastoid muscle and anterior neck: 1 = sternocleidomastoid muscle, 2 = trapezius muscle, 8 = splenius capitis, 9 = levator scapulae, 10 = middle scalene, 11 = anterior scalene, 12 = omohyoid muscle. (*Reproduced, with permission, from the University of Texas Health Science Center, Houston Medical School.*)

Contraction of the SCM has two actions. The first is **rotation of the head to the opposite side.** Thus, contraction of the right SCM will rotate the nose toward the left. The second is **lateral flexion.** Constant contraction of a single SCM will frequently result in lateral flexion to the affected side and rotation to the opposite side, sometimes called "wry neck." Co-contraction of both SCM muscles may contribute to straight flexion of the neck because the rotational movements cancel each other. However, this is not a strong action unless the neck is flexed against resistance. The **SCM** is innervated by the **spinal accessory nerve** (CN XI), which also innervates the **trapezius muscle.**

Other landmarks of the neck include the **laryngeal prominence** (Adam's apple) in the midline. This is formed by the **superior border of the thyroid cartilage.** The external jugular vein is prominent in some people. The external jugular vein forms from the posterior auricular and retromandibular veins just inferior to the ear and crosses over the SCM into the posterior triangle. Although variable, its usual course is to drain into the internal jugular before it joins with the subclavian vein. The **external jugular vein** is also a landmark for the **great auricular nerve,** which crosses the SCM as it ascends from the muscle's posterior border. Folds of the platysma muscle are observed when the skin over the neck is tensed (as in shaving). This muscle of facial expression is the most superficial muscle of the neck, and it courses just beneath the superficial fascia underlying the skin.

COMPREHENSION QUESTIONS

[38.1] A 2-year-old girl is diagnosed with torticollis involving the right SCM. Which of the following describes the most likely anatomical change?

    A. Head flexed forward in the midline

    B. Head rotated to the right

    C. Head rotated to the left

    D. Head extended in the midline plane

[38.2] A 24-year-old football player receives a blow to the left skull, and the team physician finds weakness of the left SCM. Which of the following associated findings is most likely to be seen in this patient?

    A. Weakness of the masseter muscle

    B. Decreased sensation of the ipsilateral face

    C. Decreased tearing from the ipsilateral eye

    D. Weakness of the trapezius muscle

[38.3] A clinician is palpating the anterior neck of a patient who has been involved in a motor vehicle accident and notes the laryngeal prominence. Which of the following describes the anatomical structure that corresponds to this prominence?

    A. Thyroid cartilage

    B. Cricoid cartilage

    C. Hyoid bone

    D. First tracheal ring

Answers

[38.1]   **C.** With torticollis, the SCM is shortened, leading to the head being rotated toward the contralateral side.

[38.2]   **D.** The SCM and the trapezius muscle are innervated by the spinal accessory nerve (CN XI), which is at risk in the posterior triangle of the neck.

[38.3]   **A.** The laryngeal prominence is produced by the superior border of the thyroid cartilage.

ANATOMY PEARLS

❖ The anterior neck contains structures that lie anterior to the trapezius muscle.

❖ The SCM divides the anterior neck into anterior and posterior triangles.

❖ Contraction of the SCM causes rotation of the head to the opposite side and lateral flexion.

❖ The laryngeal prominence in the midline is formed by the superior border of the thyroid cartilage

REFERENCES

Moore KL, Dalley AF. Clinically Oriented Anatomy, 5th ed. Baltimore, MD: Lippincott Williams & Wilkins, 2006:1052–8.

Netter FH. Atlas of Human Anatomy, 4th ed. Philadelphia, PA: Saunders/Elsevier, 2006:plates 28, 127.

Snell RS. Clinical Anatomy by Regions, 8th ed. Baltimore, MD: Lippincott Williams & Wilkins, 2008:735–42.

A 67-year-old man is noted to be coughing up bright red blood for a period of 1 week. He denies exposure to tuberculosis but has smoked one pack of cigarettes per day for 30 years. On examination, his lungs are clear. Palpation of the supraclavicular regions shows a hard nontender irregular mass on the left side.

◆ **What is the most likely diagnosis?**

◆ **What is the anatomical explanation for this particular mass?**

ANSWERS TO CASE 39: METASTATIC SCALENE NODE

Summary: A 67-year-old man who has smoked cigarettes for 30 years has a 1-week history of hemoptysis. Palpation of the supraclavicular regions shows a hard nontender irregular mass on the left side.

◆ **Most likely diagnosis:** Lung cancer with a left-side supraclavicular metastatic node

◆ **Anatomical explanation for this particular mass:** Lymphatic drainage through the thoracic duct to the left brachiocephalic vein

CLINICAL CORRELATION

This smoker complains of hemoptysis, the coughing of bright red blood for 1-week duration. This is very suspicious for lung cancer. In addition, he has a hard irregular mass in the left supraclavicular region. This is most likely malignant metastasis to lymph nodes in this area. Because lymph draining the abdomen, thorax, and lower extremities is directed through the thoracic duct into the left subclavian vein, the most common location of supraclavicular node involvement is the left side.

APPROACH TO THE NECK: LYMPHATICS

Objectives

1. Be able to describe general patterns of lymphatic drainage in the body.
2. Be able to distinguish lymphatic flow through the supraclavicular nodes from flow through other nodes in the neck.

Definitions

Hemoptysis: Coughing up blood.
Palpation: Technique of physical examination that uses the hands.
Metastasis: Spread of disease from one part of the body to another, usually used to describe the spread of cancer cells.

DISCUSSION

The lymphatic system complements the venous system as a pathway for return of serum constituents to the heart. Blood flows from the lungs to the periphery by the pumping action of the heart. In the closed vascular system, the venous system forms from the capillaries, the vessels with the smallest diameter. The blood is drained into increasingly larger veins as it is transported back to the heart and lungs. However, not all constituents of the extracellular fluid are captured into the venous system. A secondary pathway is through the lymphatic system. These fine vessels form from plexuses in tissues and, like veins, form vessels of increasing diameter. Unlike veins, however, the lymphatic vessels are not continuous channels. Instead, they are interrupted by **lymph nodes,** which contain dense aggregations of white blood cells.

In general, **lymphatics from below the diaphragm** on both sides of the body drain into the **cisterna chyli** and then to the **thoracic duct.** This is a particularly important pathway for fat droplets that are absorbed from the gastrointestinal tract after a meal. The thoracic duct ascends in the posterior mediastinum to drain into the venous system at the junction between the **left subclavian and internal jugular veins.** Above the diaphragm, including the head and neck, lymphatics on the left side also drain into the thoracic duct. On the **right side,** the vessels drain into the smaller right lymphatic duct, which drains variably into the **right subclavian vein.**

In the neck, **lymphatic vessels flow from superficial to deep, paralleling the major veins.** Several clusters of lymph nodes have been distinguished and divided into superficial and deep groups. In general, flow is from superior to inferior and from superficial to deep. However, the inferior deep group, which lies along the inferior portion of the internal jugular and subclavian veins, also drains the upper extremity, thorax, and abdomen.

The **lymphatic system is important for understanding the spread of cancer** (Figure 39-1). Unlike veins, the contractile force of the heart exerts no hydrostatic pressure in lymphatic vessels. **Lymph moves by compression**

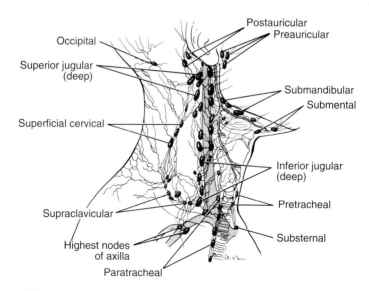

Figure 39-1. Lymphatics of the neck. (*Reproduced, with permission, from Lindner HH. Clinical Anatomy. East Norwalk, CT: Appleton & Lange, 1989:156.*)

from surrounding tissues. Few lymphatic vessels have valves, so flow is highly variable. Transformed cells from one tissue can migrate through the lymphatics to adjacent tissues. Tumor cells will frequently proliferate within lymph nodes and cause the nodes to enlarge. In the neck, the supraclavicular nodes are frequently referred to as the **sentinel nodes** because their enlargement can be the first sign of cancer originating in the thorax or abdomen.

COMPREHENSION QUESTIONS

[39.1] A 57-year-old man is diagnosed with colon cancer. He is noted to have a probable metastatic mass in the neck at the thoracic duct. Where is the metastasis likely to be located?

   A. Right supraclavicular region
   B. Right subclavicular region
   C. Left supraclavicular region
   D. Left subclavicular area

[39.2] A 65-year-old woman is noted to have cancer of the vulva. It is noted that the cancer has spread to the lymph nodes in the femoral triangle. Which of the following best describes the location of the lymph nodes?

   A. Immediately lateral to the femoral nerve
   B. Immediately medial to the femoral nerve
   C. Immediately medial to the femoral artery
   D. Immediately medial to the femoral vein
   E. Immediately lateral to the femoral vein

[39.3] What is the mechanism that propels lymph through the lymphatic vessels?

   A. Cardiac contractility
   B. Gravity
   C. Peristalsis
   D. Compression

Answers

[39.1]   **C.** The thoracic duct drains into the left subclavian vein. Malignant metastasis is often diverted to the supraclavicular nodes, where it proliferates.

[39.2]   **D.** The relations of the structures in the groin can be remembered by the mnemonic NAVEL: Nerve, Artery, Vein, Empty space, Lymph node.

[39.3]   **D.** Compression is the primary way that lymph moves through the lymphatic vessels.

ANATOMY PEARLS

 Lymphatic vessels are not continuous channels but are interrupted by lymph nodes, which contain dense aggregations of white blood cells (lymphocytes).

 In general, lymphatics from below the diaphragm on both sides of the body drain into the cisterna chyli and then to the thoracic duct.

 The lymph ascends in the posterior mediastinum to drain into the venous system at the junction between the left brachiocephalic and internal jugular veins.

REFERENCES

Moore KL, Dalley AF. Clinically Oriented Anatomy, 5th ed. Baltimore, MD: Lippincott Williams & Wilkins, 2006:181, 1108–14.

Netter FH. Atlas of Human Anatomy, 4th ed. Philadelphia, PA: Saunders/Elsevier, 2006: plate 72.

Snell RS. Clinical Anatomy by Regions, 8th ed. Baltimore, MD: Lippincott Williams & Wilkins, 2008:754–7.

A 28-year-old woman at 19 weeks of pregnancy complains of acute onset of numbness of the right cheek and drooping of the right face that occurred over 1 hour. She denies trauma to the head. On examination, the patient has difficulty closing her right eyelid, and her right nasolabial fold is smoother than on the left. She also is drooling from the right side of her mouth. The remainder of the neurological examination is normal.

◆ **What is the most likely diagnosis?**

◆ **What is the anatomical mechanism for this condition?**

ANSWERS TO CASE 40: BELL PALSY

Summary: A 28-year-old woman at 19 weeks of pregnancy complains of acute onset of numbness of the right cheek and drooping of the right face. She denies trauma to the head. On examination, the patient has difficulty closing her right eyelid and has blunting of the right nasolabial fold. The remainder of the neurological examination is normal.

◆ **Most likely diagnosis:** Bell palsy (idiopathic seventh cranial nerve palsy)

◆ **Anatomical mechanism for this condition:** Dysfunction of the peripheral portion of the seventh cranial nerve

CLINICAL CORRELATION

Bell palsy is an idiopathic form of facial nerve paralysis that usually manifests as sudden onset of unilateral facial weakness. The peripheral portion of the facial nerve (CN VII) is affected, which may lead to loss of taste to one side of the tongue, weakness of the orbicularis oculi muscle (inability to close one's eyes), and weakness of the orbicularis oris muscle (inability to purse the lips). The upper and lower portions of the face are affected, which is consistent with a peripheral neuropathy. In contrast, lower facial weakness alone may indicate an upper motor neuron lesion. Maximal weakness usually evolves over several hours and resolves by 1 week. Although patients may experience a sensation of facial numbness, there is generally no sensory loss. Pregnancy seems to increase the incidence of Bell palsy. Keeping the eye moist and protected is an important part of therapy. The eye is vulnerable to dryness due to impaired blinking. Damage to the intracranial course of parasympathetic fibers in the greater petrosal nerve may also contribute to decreased stimulation of the lacrimal gland. Oral corticosteroid therapy may help hasten the recovery. Full recovery almost always occurs.

APPROACH TO THE FACIAL NERVE

Objectives

1. Be able to describe the course of the facial nerve (CN VII).
2. Be able to list the functional components of the facial nerve.

Definitions

Bell palsy: Idiopathic palsy of peripheral CN VII leading to ipsilateral facial weakness.

Chorda tympani: Small branch of the facial nerve that supplies taste receptors in the anterior two-thirds of the tongue.

Upper motor neuron: Neurons that conduct information from motor areas of the brain to the spinal cord. The lower motor neurons project from gray matter in the spinal cord to peripheral muscle.

Vidian nerve: Nerve of the pterygoid canal.

Branchiomeric muscle: Skeletal muscle derived from one of the branchial arches. In general, this muscle is innervated by cranial nerves.

DISCUSSION

The **facial nerve (CN VII)** originates from the **lateral surface of the caudal pons,** at the **cerebellopontine junction.** There are two roots to the nerve, the large branchiomeric motor root and the small nervus intermedius, which contains sensory and visceral motor fibers. The **facial nerve runs laterally with the vestibulocochlear nerve (CN VIII)** to enter the internal acoustic meatus (Figure 40-1). The meatus is sometimes described as having four quadrants. The facial nerve goes through the anterosuperior quadrant, whereas divisions of the vestibulocochlear nerve go through the other three.

The facial nerve continues laterally until it reaches the bony labyrinth of the inner ear. At this point, the main trunk bends sharply in a posterior direction to enter the **facial canal of the temporal bone.** The bend is called the **genu.** The fibers comprising the greater petrosal nerve arise from the genu and course

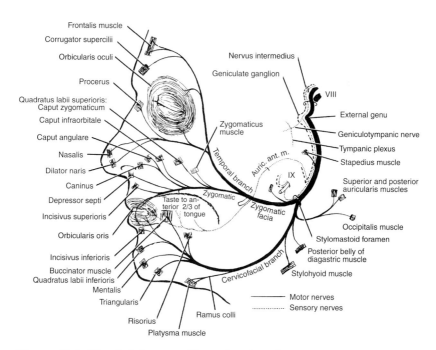

Figure 40-1. The facial nerve. (*Reproduced, with permission, from Lindner HH. Clinical Anatomy. East Norwalk, CT: Appleton & Lange, 1989:49.*)

anteriorly (described further below). Also located at the genu is the **geniculate ganglion,** the cluster of sensory cell bodies that course in the facial nerve.

The facial nerve passes through the facial canal as it courses posteriorly within the **medial wall of the tympanic cavity inferior to the lateral semicircular canal.** As the canal reaches the posterior wall of the tympanic cavity, it turns inferiorly, giving off two notable branches, described below. The nerve exits the cranium through the **stylomastoid foramen,** located between the styloid and mastoid processes.

The **facial nerve** then courses anteriorly **through the parotid gland** and splits the gland into superficial and deep lobes. The nerve diverges in variable patterns to form **five major branches** that supply the muscles of facial expression. These are the **temporal, zygomatic, buccal, mandibular, and cervical branches.** There is also a smaller posterior auricular branch that supplies the extra-auricular muscles. Sensory nerves may innervate a small patch of skin on the posterior surface of the auricle.

The **greater petrosal nerve** emerges from the **geniculate ganglion** and courses anteriorly through a small canal. It emerges through a small hiatus into the middle cranial fossa and continues anteriorly in a groove directed toward the foramen lacerum. The nerve then passes through a tunnel in the cartilage filling the foramen or through a canal in nearby bone. After exiting the basal surface of the skull posterior to the medial pterygoid plate of the sphenoid bone, the nerve heads anteriorly through the pterygoid (Vidian) canal. The pterygoid canal courses through the sphenoid bone at the base of the medial pterygoid plate. Before entering the canal, the nerve merges with the deep petrosal nerve. The newly formed nerve of the pterygoid canal (Vidian nerve) exits anteriorly into the pterygopalatine fossa. The nerve merges with the **pterygopalatine ganglion,** which is associated with branches of the **maxillary nerve (CN V2).** Sensory and sympathetic fibers pass through the ganglion and follow the branches of the maxillary nerve throughout the nasal and oral cavities. Presynaptic parasympathetic fibers synapse in the ganglion. Postsynaptic fibers project through the same nerves to innervate glands of the oral and nasal mucosa. **Visceral motor fibers innervating the lacrimal gland** also originate in the **pterygopalatine ganglion.** These fibers run from the ganglion to the infraorbital nerve (CN V2) and follow the zygomaticotemporal nerve along the lateral wall of the orbit. They then follow the lacrimal nerve (V1) to the gland. The lacrimal nerve itself is primarily sensory and innervates the periorbital skin.

As the facial nerve descends posteriorly to the tympanic cavity, two small but important branches emerge. The first is the motor branch to the **stapedius muscle.** The belly of the stapedius is contained within the pyramid. Its tendon emerges through the apex of the pyramid to attach to the body of the stapes. Contraction of the stapedius dampens the vibration of the ossicles, thus protecting against loud sounds. The second branch in this region is the **chorda tympani.** It branches from the motor trunk before it exits from the stylomastoid foramen and enters the tympanic cavity through a small canal in the posterior wall. It then runs anterolaterally, deep to the tympanic membrane. As it does so, it runs between the vertical processes of the incus and malleus. The chorda tympani courses anteriorly and inferiorly through the temporal bone and emerges from the basal surface of the skull through the petrotympanic fissure. The nerve then courses through the infratemporal fossa along the superficial surface of the medial pterygoid muscle before joining with the lingual nerve. Sensory fibers in the chorda tympani course with branches of the lingual nerve to supply **taste receptors in the anterior two-thirds of the tongue.** Presynaptic parasympathetic fibers synapse in the **submandibular ganglion.** Postsynaptic fibers supply the **submandibular and sublingual salivary glands.**

In addition to its complex branching pattern, the facial nerve has many functional components. To summarize, the facial nerve is primarily a motor nerve that supplies branchiomeric muscles. These are primarily the **muscles of facial expression** but also include the **stapedius, stylohyoid, and posterior belly of the digastric muscle.** Another important function of the facial nerve is to supply visceral motor fibers that supply the **lacrimal gland, the submandibular and sublingual salivary glands,** and mucus-secreting **glands of the nasal and oral cavities.** The facial nerve has an important sensory component. The special sensory component that supports **taste in the anterior two-thirds of the tongue is ultimately carried by the lingual nerve.** There is a minor component of general sensation from innervation of a small patch of skin on the posterior surface of the auricle.

COMPREHENSION QUESTIONS

[40.1] A 44-year-old man complains of difficulty hearing from the right ear and headaches. He also has weakness of the facial muscles. Which of the following is the most likely explanation?

    A. Peripheral CN VII palsy
    B. Peripheral CN VIII palsy
    C. Cerebellar pontine angle lesion
    D. Trigeminal ganglion lesion

[40.2] An injury to the facial nerve (CN VII) as it leaves the stylomastoid foramen would disrupt which function?

    A. Taste to the posterior tongue
    B. Sensation to the cornea
    C. Sensation to the cheek
    D. Sensation to the anterior scalp
    E. Wrinkling the forehead

[40.3] A 33-year-old woman suffered a skull fracture that led to a unilateral facial nerve palsy. Which of the following fractures was most likely responsible?

    A. Frontal calvaria
    B. Temporal bone fracture involving the squamous part
    C. Occipital fracture
    D. Basilar fracture involving the mastoid area

Answers

[40.1]   **C.** When multiple nerves are affected, it is unlikely to be a peripheral disorder. Cranial nerves VII and VIII exit in close proximity from the pons. A schwannoma involving the cerebellopontine angle can affect both cranial nerves.

[40.2]   **E.** Wrinkling the forehead is produced by contraction of the frontalis muscle, which is innervated by the facial nerve. The facial nerve is responsible for taste in the anterior two-thirds of the tongue, but the chorda tympani emerges before the main trunk exits through the stylomastoid foramen. Sensation of the cornea and sensation to the cheek are supplied by the trigeminal nerve.

[40.3]   **D.** The basilar fracture involving the mastoid region of the temporal bone may impinge on the facial nerve as it exits the stylomastoid foramen.

ANATOMY PEARLS

 Sensory fibers in the chorda tympani course with branches of the lingual nerve to supply taste receptors in the anterior two-thirds of the tongue.

 The facial nerve supplies most of the muscles involved with facial expression but also supplies the stapedius, stylohyoid, and posterior belly of the digastric muscle.

 CN VII carries visceral motor neurons that supply the lacrimal gland, the submandibular and sublingual salivary glands, and mucus-secreting glands of the nasal and oral cavities.

REFERENCES

Moore KL, Dalley AF. Clinically Oriented Anatomy, 5th ed. Baltimore, MD: Lippincott Williams & Wilkins, 2006:933–47, 1143–46.

Netter FH. Atlas of Human Anatomy, 4th ed. Philadelphia, PA: Saunders/Elsevier, 2006: plates 25, 123.

Snell RS. Clinical Anatomy by Regions, 8th ed. Baltimore, MD: Lippincott Williams & Wilkins, 2008:732–4, 763–5.

A 35-year-old woman complains of spasms of excruciating pain of the right cheek and chin. These pain episodes last for a few seconds and are intense. She had been diagnosed with multiple sclerosis 2 years previously. She is not taking medications currently, although she previously received intravenous corticosteroid therapy. Her physician says that her problem is related to the nerve that innervates the skin of the cheek area.

◆ **What is the most likely diagnosis?**

◆ **What is the anatomical explanation for this condition?**

ANSWERS TO CASE 41: TRIGEMINAL NEURALGIA

Summary: A 35-year-old woman who has multiple sclerosis complains of excruciating spasms of pain that affect her right cheek and chin and last for a few seconds.

◆ **Most likely diagnosis:** Trigeminal neuralgia

◆ **Anatomical explanation for this condition:** Pain follows the distribution of CN V, which innervates the eyes, cheeks, and chin

CLINICAL CORRELATION

Trigeminal neuralgia (tic douloureux) is among the most excruciating types of pain seen by clinicians, so intense it will cause the patient to wince. This young woman complains of several seconds of intense spasmodic pain of the right cheek and chin. Her history of multiple sclerosis is important because trigeminal neuralgia is relatively common in this group of patients. The character of the pain excludes some of the other common etiologies of the head or facial pain such as migraine headache (usually throbbing unilateral pain with orbital involvement) or tension headache (band-like constricting pain from the temples to the occiput bilaterally). She has no history of herpes simplex virus, which can also affect CN V. CN V has three branches of sensory distribution. Treatment includes carbamazepine or baclofen and, in severe cases, trigeminal nerve ablation.

APPROACH TO TRIGEMINAL NERVE

Objectives

1. Be able to relate the dermatomes of the face to the branches of the trigeminal nerve (CN V).
2. Be able to list the functions of the trigeminal nerve.

Definitions

Multiple sclerosis: Disease in which plaques in the nervous system arise because of the proliferation of fibrous connective tissue or glial cells. Sclerosis in general refers to hardening of the tissue, as in atherosclerosis, or hardening of the arteries.

Baclofen: Muscle relaxing drug that acts through type b γ-amino butyric acid ($GABA_b$) receptors.

Carbamazepine: Centrally acting anticonvulsive drug of unknown action.

DISCUSSION

The **trigeminal nerve** exits the brain from the **lateral surface of the pons.** The sensory fibers arise as a large root. Motor fibers to the **muscles of mastication** usually arise as a separate smaller root. The nerve courses on the lateral surface of the sphenoid bone deep to the cavernous sinus. The cell bodies of the sensory nerves form the **trigeminal ganglion** along the medial wall of the middle cranial fossa. Three large nerves emerge from the ganglion: the **ophthalmic, maxillary, and mandibular divisions** of the trigeminal nerve (Figure 41-1).

Branches of these nerves supply general sensation to the face and anterior scalp. The posterior scalp is supplied by cervical spinal nerves. The **ophthalmic nerve** supplies the dermatome that courses superiorly to the horizontal midline of the orbit. It also supplies the midline region of the nose. The **maxillary nerve** supplies the region over the maxilla, inferior to the orbit, including the lateral surface of the nose and the upper lip. A small band extends superiorly over the zygomatic arch and temporalis muscle. The mandibular division supplies a band of skin running superiorly over the temporalis muscle. The major branches of the ophthalmic nerve that supply the skin are the supraorbital and supratrochlear nerves, which supply skin of the forehead and anterior scalp. The nasociliary nerve supplies the skin over the medial nose through the external nasal branch of the anterior ethmoidal nerve. The maxillary nerve innervates the skin primarily through the infraorbital nerve. More laterally, the **zygomaticofacial and zygomaticotemporal nerves** also contribute. The branches of the mandibular nerve that innervate the skin are the auriculotemporal superiorly and the mental nerve (a branch of the inferior alveolar) inferiorly. The buccal nerve supplies skin over the cheek. This nerve also innervates buccal mucosa in the oral cavity. Although its branches pass through the buccinator, they do not provide motor innervation. The **buccinator** is supplied by the buccal branch of the **facial nerve (CN VII).**

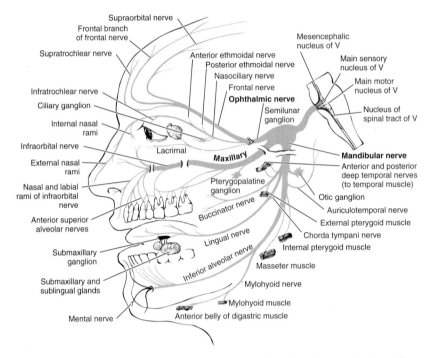

Figure 41-1. The trigeminal nerve. (*Reproduced, with permission, from Waxman SG. Clinical Neuroanatomy, 25th ed. New York: McGraw-Hill, 2003:112.*)

COMPREHENSION QUESTIONS

[41.1] A 56-year-old man had a stroke. Among other symptoms, a marked deficit in bite strength was observed on the affected side, indicating weakness in the muscles of mastication. Which of the following muscles is also innervated by the same nerve?

A. Orbicularis oculi
B. Platysma
C. Anterior belly of digastric
D. Stylohyoid
E. Superior belly of omohyoid

[41.2] A 45-year-old woman who has diabetes has developed shingles involving the right cornea. Through which nerve did the varicella virus most likely travel to the cornea?

A. CN II
B. CN III
C. CN V
D. CN VII

[41.3–41.6] Match the following divisions (A–C) to the branches [41.3–41.6].

    A. CN V1
    B. CN V2
    C. CN V3

[41.3] Auriculotemporal nerve

[41.4] Lacrimal nerve

[41.5] Supraorbital nerve

[41.6] Infraorbital nerve

Answers

[41.1] **C.** The anterior belly of digastric is innervated by CN V3, as are the muscles of mastication. The platysma and orbicularis oculi muscles are supplied by CN VII.

[41.2] **C.** The trigeminal nerve supplies sensory innervation to the cornea. Herpes simplex infections or varicella virus infections involving the face may travel through CN V to the cornea and endanger vision.

[41.3] **C.** CN V3 supplies the auriculotemporal, buccal, and mental nerves.

[41.4] **A.** CN V1 supplies the lacrimal, supraorbital, and supra- and infratrochlear nerves.

[41.5] **A.** CN V1 supplies the lacrimal, supraorbital, and supra- and infratrochlear nerves.

[41.6] **B.** CN V2 supplies the infraorbital and zygomaticotemporal nerves.

ANATOMY PEARLS

 The trigeminal nerve exits the brain from the lateral surface of the pons.

 The trigeminal nerve is comprised of three divisions: ophthalmic, maxillary, and mandibular.

 Branches of these nerves supply general sensation to the face and anterior scalp. The posterior scalp is supplied by cervical spinal nerves.

REFERENCES

Moore KL, Dalley AF. Clinically Oriented Anatomy, 5th ed. Baltimore, MD: Lippincott Williams & Wilkins, 2006:939–45, 1139–42.

Netter FH. Atlas of Human Anatomy, 4th ed. Philadelphia, PA: Saunders/Elsevier, 2006: plates 24, 122.

Snell RS. Clinical Anatomy by Regions, 8th ed. Baltimore, MD: Lippincott Williams & Wilkins, 2008:727–9, 759–62.

A 38-year-old male presents to the emergency room with complaints of a persistent headache and problems with his left eye. He has no known medical problems, and his headache is slightly improved with ibuprofen. He denies having any previous problems with his vision. On exam, he is noted to have a left eye with ptosis, dilated pupil, and displacement "down and out." The remainder of the exam is normal. An MRI shows an aneurysm of the circle of Willis.

◆ **Given the physical exam, what ocular muscles are likely not to have been affected?**

◆ **Which nerve is likely to have been affected?**

ANSWERS TO CASE 42: OCULOMOTOR NERVE PALSY

Summary: A 38-year-old healthy male with new onset left eye findings of ptosis, dilated pupil, and displacement of eye "down and out."

◆ **Ocular muscles not involved:** Superior oblique and lateral rectus

◆ **Nerve affected:** Oculomotor nerve (CN III)

CLINICAL CORRELATION

A patient with the finding of ptosis, dilated pupil, and displacement of the eye "down and out" is most consistent with oculomotor nerve palsy. The oculomotor nerve is the third of 12 paired cranial nerves and originates from the midbrain. It controls most eye movements, constriction of the pupil, and keeping the eyelid up. The "down and out" displacement of the eye occurs from the unopposed action of the lateral rectus and superior oblique. The superior oblique muscle is innervated by the trochlear nerve (CN IV), and the lateral rectus muscle is innervated by the abducens nerve (CN VI). An oculomotor nerve palsy may be caused by an aneurysm, compression, infection, infarction, or tumor.

APPROACH TO EXTRAOCULAR MUSCLES OF THE ORBIT

Objectives

1. Be able to name the seven extraocular eye muscles of each orbit, their attachments, actions, and innervation.
2. Be able to describe how each of these muscles is optimally tested in a clinical setting.
3. Be able to describe the presentation of a patient with injury to each of the nerves innervating these muscles.

Definitions

Ptosis: Drooping or partial closure of the upper eyelid.
Nerve palsy: Partial or incomplete paralysis.
Aneurysm: Dilatation of the wall of an artery due to an acquired or congenital condition.

DISCUSSION

The extraocular muscles of the orbit are the levator palpebrae superioris, four rectus (superior, inferior, lateral, and medial), and two oblique (superior and inferior) muscles. All of the extraocular muscles originate from the apex of the pyramidal shaped orbit near the optic canal, except the inferior oblique muscle, which arises from the anterior orbital floor. All but the levator palpebrae superioris attach directly to the eyeball, and are concerned with its movement. Rarely do any of the six muscles attaching directly to the eyeball move the eyeball independently from the other muscles, though their individual actions are typically described. Their attachments, actions, and innervation are listed in Table 42-1 and illustrated in Figure 42-1.

The **levator palpebrae superioris** muscle originates from the posterior orbit and attaches to the skin and tarsal plate of the upper eyelid, which it elevates. It is opposed by the superior portion of the orbicularis oculi muscle. It contains smooth muscle fibers forming the **superior tarsal** muscle that is innervated by sympathetic nerve fibers during fright or startle responses.

Table 42-1
EXTRAOCULAR MUSCLES OF THE ORBIT

MUSCLE	ORIGIN	INSERTION	ACTION	INNERVATION
Superior oblique	Posterior orbit	Posterosuperior sclera	Depresses and abducts the eye	CN IV
Inferior oblique	Anterior orbital floor	Posteroinferior sclera	Elevates and abducts the eye	CN III
Superior rectus	The common tendinous ring	The anterior portion of sclera	Elevates and adducts	CN III
Inferior rectus	The common tendinous ring	The anterior portion of sclera	Depresses and adducts	CN III
Lateral rectus	The common tendinous ring	The anterior portion of sclera	Abducts	CN VI
Medial rectus	The common tendinous ring	The anterior portion of sclera	Adducts	CN III

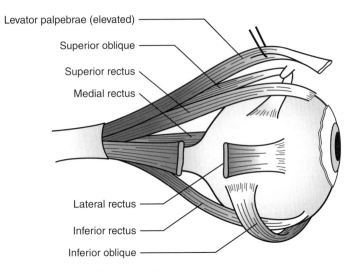

Levator palpebrae (elevated)
Superior oblique
Superior rectus
Medial rectus
Lateral rectus
Inferior rectus
Inferior oblique

Figure 42-1. Diagram of eye muscles.

The **superior oblique** muscle originates anatomically from the posterior apex of the orbit, and passes anteriorly to the **trochlea,** a pulley-like fibrous ring at the superior-medial margin on the orbit. The trochlea is the functional origin of this muscle. Its tendon passes through the trochlea to insert on posterosuperior portion of the sclera. Upon contraction, it pulls the posterior portion of the eyeball anteriorly and medially. Thus **the pupil is turned down and out.** The **inferior oblique** muscle originates from the anteromedial floor of the orbit, thus simulating the portion of the superior oblique between the trochlea and insertion. It inserts into the posteroinferior sclera, and therefore opposes the action of the superior oblique. It will turn the pupil of the eye up and out. The two oblique muscles also produce extorsion or lateral rotation of the eyeball.

The four rectus muscles (superior, inferior, lateral, and medial) all originate from a common tendinous ring surrounding the optic canal and a portion of the superior orbital fissure in the posterior orbit. Each inserts on the anterior half of the sclera on that portion of the eyeball according to their name. Thus the lateral rectus inserts on the anterolateral sclera. Note superior and inferior rectus will also turn the eyeball in or adduct the pupil. The superior and inferior recti muscle also produce intorsion or medial rotation of the eyeball.

For the sake of clarity, the following descriptions for muscle testing are for **only the right eye.** For optimal testing of the extraocular muscles, the axis of the muscle is placed parallel with the axis of muscle pull. With the eyeball (pupil) abducted, the superior and inferior recti are in line with their pull, and their action on the eyeball is almost purely elevation and depression respectively. For the superior and inferior oblique muscles, adduction of the eyeball (pupil) places the axis of the muscle in line with its pull (remember the functional origin of the superior oblique is the trochlea). Thus the eyeball (pupil) is depressed and elevated for these two muscles respectively. The lateral and medial recti are tested by simply adducting or abducting the eyeball (pupil) respectively. (see Figure 42-2).

If the **oculomotor nerve** (CN III) is injured as in this case, the pupil of the affected eye will be turned down and out (because of the unopposed action of the superior oblique and lateral rectus muscle. The pupil will also be dilated due to loss of the parasympathetic innervation to the constrictor muscle of the pupil. Loss of the **trochlear nerve,** though rare, results in slight adduction of the affected eye, weakness of downward gaze due to paralysis of the superior oblique, and head tilting to eliminate diplopia (double vision). Loss of **abducens nerve** (CN VI) function results in paralysis of the lateral rectus muscle, and thus the patient's affected eye will be turned in or adducted.

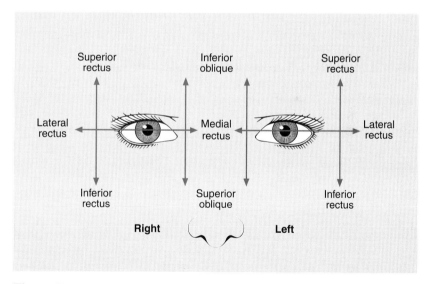

Figure 42-2. Diagram of eye muscle action.

COMPREHENSION QUESTIONS

[42.1] During a physical examination of a patient, you notice ptosis of the patient's left eye. This would indicate to you there is paralysis of which muscle?

    A. Orbicularis muscle
    B. Superior oblique muscle
    C. Inferior oblique muscle
    D. Inferior rectus muscle
    E. Levator palpebrae muscle

[42.2] While performing a physical examination, you test the function of the muscles attached to the eyeball, and thereby the integrity of their innervation. You would test the function of the superior oblique muscle by having the patient do which of the following?

    A. Look in toward the nose
    B. Look laterally
    C. Look in toward the nose and then upward
    D. Look in toward the nose and then down
    E. Look laterally and then down

[42.3] During this same physical exam, you ask the patient to look laterally with her right eye, and then upward. You have just tested the function of which muscle?

    A. Superior rectus muscle
    B. Superior oblique muscle
    C. Inferior oblique muscle
    D. Inferior rectus muscle
    E. Medial rectus muscle

Answers

[42.1]   **E.** Ptosis or drooping of the eyelid is due to paralysis of the levator palpebrae muscle. The orbicularis muscle closes the eyelid.

[42.2]   **D.** Turning the eyeball inward places the portion of the superior oblique between the trochlea and its insertion places the axis of the muscle in line with its axis of muscle pull. Because the muscle's insertion is on the posterior portion of the sclera, it will then turn the eye (pupil) down (depress).

[42.3]   **A.** Turning the eyeball out places the axis of the superior rectus muscle parallel to its pull and the muscle will then turn the eyeball upward (elevate).

ANATOMY PEARLS

 $LR_6SO_4AO_3$: lateral rectus, CN **VI**; superior oblique, CN **IV**; all others, CN **III.**

 The functional portion of the superior oblique muscle is between the trochlea and the insertion of the tendon.

 The oculomotor nerve (CN III) innervates the majority of the extraocular muscles, the sphincter muscle of the pupil, and the smooth muscle fibers of the superior tarsal muscle.

REFERENCES

Moore KL, Dalley, AF. Clinically Oriented Anatomy, 5th ed. Baltimore, MD: Lippincott Williams & Wilkins, 2006:968–72.

Netter FH. Atlas of Human Anatomy, 4th ed. Philadelphia, PA: Saunders, 2006: plates 84, 86.

Snell RS. Clinical Anatomy by Regions, 8th ed. Baltimore, MD: Lippincott Williams & Wilkins, 2008:691, 699–701.

A male infant who weighs 3500-g appears icteric on examination. The previous day, the infant was delivered vaginally by vacuum-assisted extraction because there were severe fetal heart rate decelerations. The infant's scalp has a 5-cm discolored soft tissue swelling that seems to be contained by and does not cross the sagittal or lambdoidal sutures. The mother had no prenatal or medical problems. There is no family history of bleeding disorders.

◆ **What is the most likely diagnosis?**

◆ **What is the anatomical mechanism for the condition?**

ANSWERS TO CASE 43: CEPHALOHEMATOMA

Summary: On the previous day, a male infant who weighs 3500 g was born vaginally by vacuum-assisted extraction. The infant appears icteric, and his scalp has a 5-cm hematoma that is contained by and does not cross the sagittal or lambdoidal sutures.

◆ **Most likely diagnosis:** Cephalohematoma

◆ **Anatomical mechanism for the condition:** Injury to the branches of arteries supplying the lateral skull

CLINICAL CORRELATION

This 1-day-old infant was delivered with the aid of vacuum extraction and now has icterus and a discolored soft tissue mass that is contained within the sutures. This almost certainly represents a cephalohematoma. The more common caput succedaneum, which is swelling of the scalp soft tissue, is a normal response of the fetal head to the birth process. In this situation, the blood will cross over suture lines. When a soft tissue mass seems contained by suture lines, then subgaleal cephalohematoma is suspected. The hemoglobin deposited in the hematoma becomes bilirubin, which is the reason for the infant's icterus. A skull radiograph or CT scan is usually obtained to assess for skull fracture. Most of these hematomas will resolve with observation.

APPROACH TO THE SCALP AND SKULL

Objectives

1. Be able to define the layers of the scalp.
2. Be able to describe the structure of cranial sutures.

Definitions

Major sutures of the skull: The sagittal suture runs along the midline of the skull between the two parietal bones. The lambdoidal suture runs left to right posteriorly and separates the two parietal bones from the occipital bone. The coronal suture has the same course anteriorly and separates the frontal bone from the two parietal bones.

Hematoma: Pool of blood that accumulates in a tissue or space, usually clotted.

Bilirubin: Bile salt that is formed from the breakdown of hemoglobin by the liver. It usually accumulates in the gallbladder and is excreted into the small bowel to aid in digestion. High levels of bilirubin in the blood give the skin and sclera of the eyes a yellowish tint (jaundice).

Icteric: Yellowish appearance of jaundice, in this case due to the local breakdown of bilirubin in the blood that has accumulated in the hematoma.

Caput succedaneum: Edematous swelling of the superficial scalp due to the normal trauma of the birth process that resolves within 2 to 3 days.

DISCUSSION

The scalp is the unit of tissue that covers the calvaria. The tissue is composed of **five layers** and can be remembered by the acronym **SCALP** (Figure 43-1). Most superficial is the **skin,** which includes the dermis and the superficial fascia. Deep to that is a layer of dense **connective tissue** that binds tightly to the skin. The next

Figure 43-1. The layers of the scalp: 1 = skin, 2 = connective tissue, 3 = aponeurosis, 4 = loose connective tissue, 5 = periosteum, 8 = outer table of calvaria, 9 = diploe, 10 = inner table of calvaria, 11 = endocranium. (*Reproduced, with permission, from the University of Texas Health Science Center, Houston Medical School.*)

layer is the **aponeurosis** of the occipitofrontalis muscle (galea aponeurotica). These three layers adhere tightly and move together as a unit. The fourth layer is one of **loose connective tissue.** The fifth layer is the **periosteum,** which covers the bone itself. The periosteum adheres tightly to the bone, especially in the region of the cranial sutures. The flexibility of the loose connective tissue allows the more superficial layers to move over the periosteum. In infants, the periosteum is adherent to the sutures.

The blood vessels that supply the scalp are from branches of the **internal and external carotid arteries. Anteriorly,** these are the **supraorbital and supratrochlear arteries which are derived from the internal carotid.** More **laterally and posteriorly,** the scalp is supplied by branches of the **external carotid arteries.** These include the **superficial temporal arteries,** which ascend in front of the auricle, and the **occipital** and **posterior auricular arteries,** which ascend posterior to the auricle. **The arteries of the scalp are highly anastomotic.** Therefore, after a laceration, blood may pulse from both ends of the cut artery.

The **nerves of the scalp anteriorly** are from the **first and third divisions of the trigeminal nerve. Medially,** the **supraorbital and supratrochlear nerves** supply sensory innervation. Laterally, the **auriculotemporal nerve** provides sensory innervation. The posterior scalp is supplied medially by the posterior primary rami of cervical spinal nerves (C2, as the greater occipital nerve, and C3). Laterally, the skin is supplied by anterior primary rami that form the cervical plexus, in particular the **lesser occipital and posterior auricular nerves.**

Trauma to the scalp can damage blood vessels and, hence, cause a **hematoma.** The hematoma may spread within the same layer. Blood in the superficial fascia will migrate a little more slowly because of the septa within the subcutaneous fascia. In newborn infants, hematomas in this layer commonly result from the trauma of movement through the birth canal. Likewise, scalp trauma such as that induced by a suction-assisted delivery may occasionally injure the **arteries within the periosteum, leading to accumulation of blood between the periosteum and the bone.** Because the periosteum in infants adheres to the sutures, spread is impeded. A subcutaneous hematoma will cross sutures, but a subperiosteal hematoma will not. In adults, the **loose connective layer** is called the danger space because infection can easily migrate to the **periorbital space.** This is a dangerous condition because of the potential for spread into the cranium through the **cavernous sinus.**

COMPREHENSION QUESTIONS

[43.1] Which of the following best describes the layers of scalp?

    A. Skin, aponeurosis, dense connective tissue, periosteum

    B. Skin, loose connective tissue, aponeurosis, periosteum

    C. Skin, dense connective tissue, aponeurosis, loose connective tissue, periosteum

    D. Skin, aponeurosis, loose connective tissue, muscle, periosteum

[43.2] A 65-year-old woman complains of severe pain of the right side of the head. A vascular surgeon takes a biopsy of the artery deep to the temporalis muscle. Which of the following vessels did the surgeon most likely biopsy?

    A. Middle meningeal artery

    B. External carotid artery

    C. Ophthalmic artery

    D. Deep temporal artery

[43.3] A neurologist uses a pin to test the sensation to a 26-year-old man's scalp just near the hair line anteriorly. Which of the following nerves provides the innervation to the scalp in this region?

    A. CN V

    B. CN VII

    C. CN X

    D. Spinal nerve C2

Answers

[43.1] **C.** The layers of the scalp can be remembered by the mnemonic SCALP: Skin, Connective tissue, Aponeurosis, Loose connective tissue, Periosteum.

[43.2] **D.** The temporal artery is deep to the temporalis muscle and sometimes is associated with inflammation (temporal arteritis). Temporal arteritis or giant cell arteritis is associated with headache and multiple joint pain.

[43.3] **A.** The anterior scalp is innervated by CN V, whereas the posterior scalp is innervated by spinal nerve C2.

ANATOMY PEARLS

❖ The layers of the scalp can be remembered by the mnemonic **SCALP**: **S**kin, **C**onnective tissue, **A**poneurosis, **L**oose connective tissue, **P**eriosteum.

❖ The blood vessels that supply the scalp are from branches of the internal and external carotid arteries.

❖ The sensory innervation of the scalp is by the trigeminal nerve: anteriorly by the supraorbital and supratrochlear nerves; laterally by the auriculotemporal nerve. The posterior scalp is innervated by spinal nerves C2 and C3. Spinal nerve C1 does not have a sensory component.

❖ Infants who undergo trauma, such as that induced by a suction-assisted delivery, may experience damage to the arteries within the periosteum and develop a subperiosteal hematoma.

REFERENCES

Bickley LS, Szilagyi PG. Bate's Guide to the Physical Examination and History Taking, 8th ed, Philadelphia, PA: Lippincott Williams & Wilkins, 2003:667–8.

Moore KL, Dalley AF. Clinically Oriented Anatomy, 5th ed. Baltimore, MD: Lippincott Williams & Wilkins, 2006:906–8.

Netter FH. Atlas of Human Anatomy, 4th ed. Philadelphia, PA: Saunders/Elsevier, 2006: plates 12, 23.

Snell RS. Clinical Anatomy by Regions, 8th ed. Baltimore, MD: Lippincott Williams & Wilkins, 2008:722–6.

A 15-year-old boy was the pitcher for his little league baseball team when he was hit by a line drive to the right temple area. He lost consciousness briefly but woke up after about 45 seconds and had no neurological deficits. He was taken to the emergency room and seemed to be in good condition. Four hours later, while being observed, he complained of an increasing headache and had a seizure. On examination, the patient's right pupil appeared dilated and reacted sluggishly to light. The emergency physician is concerned about increased intracranial pressure.

◆ **What is the most likely diagnosis?**

◆ **What is the anatomical explanation for this condition?**

ANSWERS TO CASE 44: EPIDURAL HEMATOMA

Summary: A 15-year-old boy was hit by a baseball to the right temple area. He lost consciousness briefly and had a lucid interval. Four hours later, he developed an increasing headache, a dilated and sluggish right pupil, and had a seizure, consistent with increased intracranial pressure.

◆   **Most likely diagnosis:** Epidural hematoma resulting in increased intracranial pressure

◆   **Anatomical explanation for this condition:** Disruption of a branch of the middle meningeal artery, which causes a growing hematoma between the dura and cranium and puts pressure on the underlying brain

CLINICAL CORRELATION

This 15-year-old baseball player underwent significant blunt trauma to the right temple area by a baseball. He had a brief loss of consciousness, likely due to the concussion of the baseball. After waking up, he had no neurological deficits; however, after 4 hours, there were signs of increased intracranial pressure. The most likely explanation is disruption of the middle meningeal artery, which underlies the temporal bone. Over time, the hematoma formed, putting pressure on the underlying brain tissue. The ipsilateral pupil was affected due to compression of the oculomotor nerve (CN III) by the temporal lobe of the brain. This scenario of a loss of consciousness followed by a lucid interval and a second loss of consciousness is very typical for epidural hematoma. Because this is arterial bleeding, rapid expansion of the hematoma is typical. Emergent cerebral decompression and surgical control of the bleeding is paramount.

APPROACH TO MENINGES AND ARTERIAL SUPPLY TO BRAIN

Objectives

1.   Be able to list the meningeal layers.
2.   Be able to identify the dural folds and associated dural sinuses.
3.   Be able to describe the vascular supplies to the meninges and underlying brain.

Definitions

Pachymeninx: The thick meningeal layer, that is, the dura mater.
Leptomeninx: The thin meningeal layers, that is, the arachnoid and pia maters together.

Dural sinus: Cavity filled with venous blood formed by a split in the two layers of dura mater, the periosteal and meningeal layers. Blood drains from the system of sinuses into the internal jugular vein.

Pterion: A landmark on the lateral surface of the skull formed by the junction of the frontal, parietal, temporal, and sphenoid bones. It usually has an H-shaped appearance.

DISCUSSION

As in the spinal cord, there are **three meningeal layers that cover the brain: the dura mater, arachnoid mater, and pia mater.** The **dura mater is a thick, strong membrane (pachymeninx)** that is closely apposed to the deep surface of the cranium. Immediately deep to the dura is the arachnoid layer, a thin, nearly transparent membrane that adheres to the deep surface of the dura. The arachnoid layer is separated from the brain by the **subarachnoid space, which is filled with CSF.** The **pia mater** is a thin layer attached to the surface of the brain itself. The **arachnoid and pia layers together** may be referred to as the **leptomeninges.**

The **dura mater** that covers the external surface of the brain consists of **two layers, an external periosteal layer attached to the bone and an internal meningeal layer.** The internal layer forms folds that separate the major lobes of the brain. The **falx cerebri** courses along the midline and separates the left and right cerebral hemispheres. Running at right angles, the **tentorium cerebelli** separates the two lobes of the cerebrum from the cerebellum. On the inferior surface of the tentorium is attached the small **falx cerebelli**, which also runs along the midline and partially separates the cerebellum into lobes. Another important dural infolding covers the pituitary fossa and is the called the **diaphragma sellae**.

Normally, the two dural layers are tightly apposed, but they may split to form the **dural sinuses (Figure 44-1).** The major dural sinuses are **the superior sagittal sinus,** which courses along the superior edge of the falx cerebri, and the **transverse sinus,** which courses along the posterior border of the tentorium cerebelli. The **transverse sinus** continues laterally as the **sigmoid sinus** and empties into the internal jugular vein. On the inferior surface of the falx cerebri, the **inferior sagittal sinus** continues as the straight sinus after joining the **great vein of Galen,** which drains the brain. The **superior, straight, and transverse sinuses come together at the confluence of sinuses,** a landmark on the internal surface of the occipital bone. Other important sinuses are the superior and inferior petrosal sinuses and the cavernous sinus.

The vessels that supply the dura mater are branches of the **middle meningeal artery.** This artery arises in the infratemporal fossa from the first part of the maxillary artery and enters the cranial cavity through the foramen spinosum. The artery runs within the dura mater and separates into anterior and posterior divisions. An external landmark for the middle meningeal artery

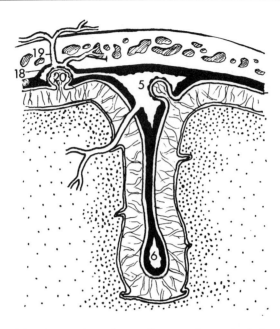

Figure 44-1. The dura and meninges: 5 = superior sagittal sinus, 6 = inferior sagittal sinus, 18 = lateral lacuna, 19 = emissary vein (connects sinuses to scalp veins), 20 = arachnoid granulation (resorption of cerebrospinal fluid). (*Reproduced, with permission, from the University of Texas Health Science Center, Houston Medical School.*)

is the **pterion, where the frontal, parietal, temporal, and sphenoid bones converge.** The vessels that supply the brain arise from the **circle of Willis** (see Case 46 for more details). This **anastomotic formation originates from the internal carotid and vertebral arteries.** The major branches tend to course along the surface of the brain and give off penetrating branches.

Head trauma can result in damage to vessels and internal bleeding. Blood accumulates in potential spaces surrounding the brain, expanding their volume, and putting pressure on the brain. The site of accumulation is characteristic of the type of vessel that is damaged. For example, rupture of the **middle meningeal artery** will lead to accumulation of blood in the **epidural potential space, between the external periosteal layer of the dura and the calvaria.** Blood from a **cerebral artery** due, for example, to a **ruptured cerebral aneurysm,** will accumulate in the **subarachnoid space.** Head trauma may result in **rupture of veins as they enter a sinus,** usually resulting in accumulation of blood in **the subdural potential space between the dural and arachnoid layers.** These veins may be cerebral veins that drain the brain or emissary veins that drain the scalp.

COMPREHENSION QUESTIONS

[44.1] A 35-year-old man developed an intracranial hemorrhage when one of the meningeal arteries ruptured. Anatomically, where is the hematoma located?

 A. Immediately superficial to the dura
 B. Immediately deep to the dura
 C. Within the subarachnoid space
 D. Within the brain parenchyma

[44.2] A 1-month-old infant is seen in the emergency department due to lethargy and seizures. After careful questioning, it was discovered that the infant was shaken before the change in mental status. Which vessels are most likely to be injured?

 A. Meningeal arteries
 B. Meningeal veins
 C. Emissary veins
 D. Middle cerebral arteries

[44.3] A 21-year-old man is brought into the emergency room after being hit in the head with a baseball bat. The neurosurgeon notes that the skull fracture and underlying hematoma seem to have occurred at the junction of the four major bones of the skull. Which of the following describes this region?

 A. Bregma
 B. Lambda
 C. Pterion
 D. Nasion

Answers

[44.1] **A.** Injuries to the meningeal arteries lead to epidural hematomas.

[44.2] **C.** Infants who are shaken are vulnerable to laceration of the emissary veins that are found below the dura. Thus, they often develop subdural hematomas.

[44.3] **C.** The pterion is a landmark of the skull where the four major bones of the skull (frontal, parietal, temporal, and sphenoidal) come together. It is also the thinnest part of the skull.

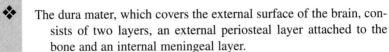

ANATOMY PEARLS

❖ The dura mater, which covers the external surface of the brain, consists of two layers, an external periosteal layer attached to the bone and an internal meningeal layer.

❖ An external landmark for the middle meningeal artery is the pterion, where the frontal, parietal, temporal, and sphenoid bones converge.

❖ The vessels that supply the dura mater are branches of the middle meningeal artery, and injuries to these vessels lead to epidural hematomas.

❖ Blood from ruptured cerebral arteries due, for example, to a ruptured cerebral aneurysm, will accumulate in the subarachnoid space.

REFERENCES

Moore KL, Dalley AF. Clinically Oriented Anatomy, 5th ed. Baltimore, MD: Lippincott Williams & Wilkins, 2006:908–21.

Netter FH. Atlas of Human Anatomy, 4th ed. Philadelphia, PA: Saunders/Elsevier, 2006:plates 100–2.

Snell RS. Clinical Anatomy by Regions, 8th ed. Baltimore, MD: Lippincott Williams & Wilkins, 2008:681–7.

A 36-year-old woman complains of pain and swelling beneath the left mandible, particularly after eating a meal. On examination, she is noted to have edema and tenderness of the left submandibular region. Palpation of her mouth reveals a 4-mm, irregular, nonmobile, hard mass in the mucosa of her mouth. She denies trauma to the region and does not have an eating disorder.

◆ **What is the most likely diagnosis?**

◆ **What is the anatomical course of the affected structure?**

ANSWERS TO CASE 45: SALIVARY STONE

Summary: A 36-year-old woman complains of pain and swelling of the left submandibular area. On examination, she has tenderness of the left submandibular salivary gland and a palpable, irregular, 4-mm mass along the floor of her mouth. She denies trauma to the region and does not have an eating disorder.

◆ **Most likely diagnosis:** Stone in the submandibular duct (sialolithiasis).

◆ **Anatomical course of the affected structure:** The submandibular salivary duct drains from the deep lobe of the submandibular gland and courses anterolaterally along the base of the tongue. Occlusion of the duct by a stone will cause secreted saliva to accumulate proximally to the stone, thus causing distention and pain.

CLINICAL CORRELATION

This 36-year-old woman has sudden onset of pain to the left submandibular area. The pain is most intense after a meal. She also complains of a "sand-like" or "gritty" sensation in her mouth. The left submandibular gland appears swollen. This is most consistent with a stone in the submandibular duct. Pain after a meal is from the accumulation of saliva proximal to the occluded duct, which stretches the duct or the capsule of the gland. Generalized swelling may be due to a secondary infection. The pathogenesis of sialolithiasis is unknown but appears to be due to lodging of a small particle in the duct, which serves as a nucleus for deposition of organic and inorganic material. The particle could be food, bacteria, or an inorganic constituent of tobacco smoke. The next diagnostic step would be examination with sialoendoscopy. Treatment would be excision of the stone under endoscopy and administration of antibiotics. If necessary, the gland would be removed surgically.

APPROACH TO SALIVARY GLANDS

Objectives

1. Be able to describe the salivary glands and the course of their ducts to the oral cavity.
2. Be able to identify structures in the floor of the mouth related to the submandibular gland.

Definitions

Caruncle: Small protuberance, or papilla.
Frenulum: Mucosal fold that extends along the midline from the floor of the mouth to the inferior surface of the tongue.

DISCUSSION

Three salivary glands form an irregular, space-filling ring around the oral cavity (Figure 45-1). The **parotid gland** lies superficial and posterior to the ramus of the mandible and inferior to the ear. The **submandibular gland** lies below the angle and the body of the mandible superficial to the mylohyoid muscle. The **sublingual gland** lies in the floor of the mouth between the mandible and the genioglossus muscle. All of the glands secrete saliva into the oral cavity through characteristic ducts. The parotid duct emerges from the anterior border of the parotid gland. The **parotid duct crosses over the masseter muscle** and pierces through the buccinator muscle to open into the oral cavity, typically at the level of the second upper molar. The **submandibular duct** forms from the deep lobe of the submandibular gland, **deep to the mylohyoid muscle.** The duct runs anteriorly on the surface of the hyoglossus muscle and opens into the oral cavity through the submandibular caruncles, just lateral to the lingual frenulum. The **sublingual glands** give rise to numerous small ducts that **empty at the base of the tongue.**

The **submandibular duct** has a close relation to several important structures in the floor of the mouth. The submandibular gland folds around the free

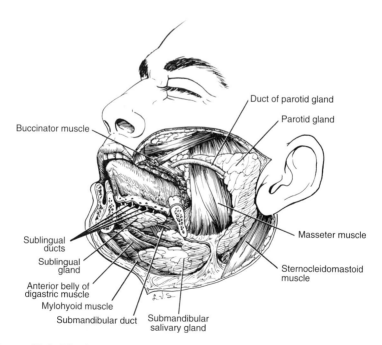

Figure 45-1. The large salivary glands. (*Reproduced, with permission, from Lindner HH. Clinical Anatomy. East Norwalk, CT: Appleton & Lange, 1989:60.*)

posterior border of the **mylohyoid muscle,** and the duct arises from the deep lobe of the gland. It courses anteriorly between the mylohyoid and hyoglossus muscles and then on the deep surface of the sublingual gland. The **hypoglossal nerve (CN XII) courses inferior to the submandibular duct** to enter the inferior surface of the genioglossus muscle. The lingual nerve descends on the surface of the medial pterygoid muscle and loops underneath the duct before innervating the anterior portion of the tongue.

COMPREHENSION QUESTIONS

[45.1] A 22-year-old male is involved in a knife fight after a soccer game. He is brought to the emergency department. An 8-cm laceration that involves the right cheek, from his right ear to near the corner of his mouth, is noted. Which of the following structures is most likely injured?

A. Parotid duct
B. Submandibular duct
C. Superficial temporal artery
D. Lingual artery
E. Mandibular branch of the facial nerve

[45.2] A 45-year-old woman is undergoing surgical resection of the salivary gland for probable cancer. After surgery, she notes that she cannot move her tongue well. Which of the following salivary glands is most likely involved in the surgery?

A. Parotid
B. Sublingual
C. Submandibular
D. Maxillary

[45.3] A 16-year-old girl is brought into the physician's office because her mother suspects an eating disorder. The patient has bilateral swelling of the cheeks that are nontender. There are multiple dental caries. She appears to be of normal weight. Which of the following is the most likely diagnosis?

A. Anorexia nervosa
B. Bulimia
C. Irritable bowel syndrome
D. Facetious hyperphagia

Answers

[45.1]   **A.** The buccal branch of the facial nerve and the parotid duct travel in the area of the cheek and can be located by a line drawn from the tragus of the ear (or the external auditory meatus) to the corner of the mouth.

[45.2]   **C.** The hypoglossal nerve courses deep to the submandibular gland, and injury to this nerve weakens or paralyzes muscles of the tongue.

[45.3]   **B.** Enlargement of the parotid glands and multiple dental caries are common in individuals who have bulimia. Affected patients may be of normal weight or even slightly overweight, and their behavior is characterized by binges of eating and inducing vomiting or use of laxatives.

REFERENCES

Marchal F, Dulguerov P. Sialolithiasis management: the state of the art. Arch Otolaryngol Head Neck Surg 2003;129:951–6.

Moore KL, Dalley AF. Clinically Oriented Anatomy, 5th ed. Baltimore, MD: Lippincott Williams & Wilkins, 2006:953–5, 1008–10.

Netter FH. Atlas of Human Anatomy, 4th ed. Philadelphia, PA: Saunders/Elsevier, 2006: plates 46, 53, 60–1.

Snell RS. Clinical Anatomy by Regions, 8th ed. Baltimore, MD: Lippincott Williams & Wilkins, 2008:787–9.

A 43-year-old man was washing his car when he suddenly complained of a severe headache and then slumped to the ground. His son, who had witnessed the episode, stated that his father grabbed his head with both hands and cried out in pain as he was falling. The son said that his father had no medical problems and exercised regularly. On examination in the emergency department, the patient was lethargic but responsive to deep pain stimuli. His pupils were dilated bilaterally and sluggishly reactive to light. CT scan of the head showed a significant intracranial hemorrhage. An angiogram demonstrated leakage of dye from the junction of the right internal carotid artery and the circle of Willis.

◆ **What is the most likely diagnosis?**

◆ **What is the clinical anatomy for this event?**

ANSWERS TO CASE 46: BERRY ANEURYSM

Summary: An otherwise healthy 43-year-old man suddenly complained of a severe headache and lost consciousness. He is lethargic, responsive to deep pain, and has bilaterally dilated and sluggishly reactive pupils. CT imaging showed a significant intracranial hemorrhage, and an angiogram demonstrated leakage of dye from the junction of the right internal carotid artery and the circle of Willis.

◆ **Most likely diagnosis:** Ruptured berry aneurysm

◆ **Clinical anatomy for this event:** Weakness of the intracranial arterial junction

CLINICAL CORRELATION

This otherwise healthy 43-year-old man had an acute and significant cerebral event. He had a severe headache quickly followed by loss of consciousness. There was no motor activity to suggest an epileptic seizure. Further, his comatose state ruled out self-limited etiologies such as syncope due to a vasovagal reaction. The cerebral imaging confirms intracranial hemorrhage. The possibilities include an arteriovenous malformation (a tangle of vessels that sometimes rupture) or a hemorrhagic stroke. The arteriogram shows leakage of dye from the junction of the internal carotid artery and the circle of Willis, strongly suggesting a berry aneurysm. The blood supply to the brain is derived from the paired internal carotid and the paired vertebral arteries. Occlusion of even one of these vessels would cause severe damage were it not for the anastomosis between these four vessels known as the circle of Willis. However, there is inherent weakness at the junction of the arteries, and an outpouching of the arterial wall, a berry aneurysm, may occur and ultimately rupture. The best treatment for such a ruptured aneurysm is surgical clip ligation. Medications such as calcium channel blockers are useful for preventing coexisting arterial vasospasm.

APPROACH TO VASCULAR SUPPLY OF BRAIN

Objectives

1. Be able to describe the course of the internal carotid and vertebral arteries.
2. Be able to list the major intracranial branches of the internal carotid and the basilar arteries.
3. Be able to identify the components of the circle of Willis.

Definitions

Angiography: Radiographic technique in which contrast medium is injected into the arterial system. X-ray images may be taken at regular intervals to follow the dye from the arterial supply through the venous drainage. Recent advances in MRI have made it possible to examine blood flow without injection of contrast medium.

Aneurysm: Disruption within the wall of an artery that fills with blood and inflates the muscular coat. The resulting dilation can exert pressure on surrounding structures and ultimately may rupture, leading to a rapid loss of blood pressure.

Syncope: Episode of fainting; a loss of consciousness not related to sleeping.

DISCUSSION

The **arterial blood supply to the brain** is derived from the **paired internal carotid** and **paired vertebral arteries.** The **internal carotid arteries** arise from the **bifurcation of the common carotid arteries** at about the level of the **superior border of the thyroid cartilage.** They are described as the direct continuation of the common carotids, have no branches in the neck, and ascend to the base of the skull, where they enter the carotid canal. The **internal carotid arteries** pass anteriorly and medially through the **cavernous sinus** to enter the cranial cavity and divide into its terminal branches, the **anterior cerebral artery** and the **middle cerebral artery.** The two anterior cerebral arteries join through the anterior communicating branch. The posterior communicating branch joins the middle cerebral with the posterior cerebral arteries.

The **vertebral arteries** are the first branches of the subclavian arteries in the root of the neck. They ascend through the **transverse foramina of vertebrae C6 to C1,** enter the cranial cavity through the **foramen magnum,** and unite to form the **basilar artery** near the junction of the pons and medulla (Figure 46-1). At the superior border of the pons, it divides into the **posterior**

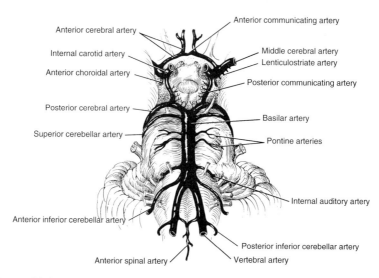

Figure 46-1. The circle of Willis. (*Reproduced, with permission, from Chusid JG. Correlative Neuroanatomy and Functional Neurology, 19th ed. East Norwalk, CT: Appleton & Lange, 1985.*)

cerebral arteries. The chief intracranial branches of the **vertebral arteries** are the **posterior inferior cerebellar arteries**. Before its terminal bifurcation, the chief branches of the basilar artery are the **anterior inferior cerebellar arteries, superior cerebellar arteries, and several pontine branches**.

The **cerebral arterial circle (of Willis)** is the major anastomosis of the cerebral vasculature. This allows for perfusion of the brain even with arterial occlusion of one or more major arteries (such as carotid insufficiency). If the occlusion develops slowly, the anastomotic vessels will expand to compensate. However, the anastomosis may not be able to compensate if the occlusion develops rapidly, as with trauma. Blockage of one cerebral artery will have characteristic effects based on the region of the brain supplied by the vessel (Figure 46-2). The **anterior cerebral artery** supplies the medial surface of the cerebrum. The **middle cerebral artery** supplies the lateral surfaces, and the

LATERAL SURFACE

MEDIAN SURFACE

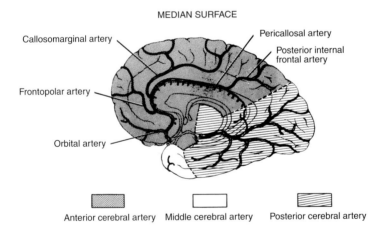

Figure 46-2. Arterial supply of the cerebral cortex. (*Reproduced, with permission, from Lindner HH. Clinical Anatomy. East Norwalk, CT:Appleton & Lange, 1989:32.*)

posterior cerebral artery supplies the inferior surface. The middle cerebral artery is occluded most often, presumably because it follows the same trajectory as the internal carotid.

COMPREHENSION QUESTIONS

[46.1] A 53-year-old man is being examined for carotid bruits. The physician would like to auscultate the internal carotid artery. At what level does the carotid artery usually bifurcate into the internal and external carotid arteries?

    A. At the level of the cricoid cartilage
    B. At the level of the thyroid cartilage
    C. At the level of sternal notch
    D. At the level of the C8 vertebra

[46.2] A 64-year-old man is diagnosed with an acute stroke. His main deficit is a partial loss of his visual field. The neurologist diagnoses a lesion of the occipital lobe. Which of the following arteries is likely to be involved?

    A. Internal carotid
    B. External carotid
    C. Middle cerebral
    D. Posterior cerebral

[46.3] A 35-year-old man complains of the worst headache of his life, grabs onto the back of his neck, and then slumps onto the floor. At the hospital, his CT findings are consistent with a subarachnoid hemorrhage. Which of the following is the most likely etiology?

    A. Carotid artery occlusion
    B. Vertebrobasilar artery occlusion
    C. Middle meningeal artery laceration
    D. Rupture of a berry aneurysm

Answers

[46.1]   **B.** The carotid artery bifurcates at the level of the thyroid cartilage.

[46.2]   **D.** The occipital lobes are supplied by the posterior cerebral arteries, which are terminal branches of the basilar artery.

[46.3]   **D.** The most common causes of subarachnoid hemorrhage are rupture of a berry aneurysm in the circle of Willis and bleeding from an arteriovenous malformation.

ANATOMY PEARLS

❖ The internal carotid arteries have no branches in the neck.
❖ The terminal branches of the internal carotid arteries are the anterior and middle cerebral arteries.
❖ The blood supply to the cerebellum is derived from the vertebrobasilar arterial system.
❖ The circle of Willis allows anastomosis of the arterial blood supply of the brain.
❖ The major arterial blood supply of the brain is from the internal carotid and vertebral arteries.

REFERENCES

Moore KL, Dalley AF. Clinically Oriented Anatomy, 5th ed. Baltimore, MD: Lippincott Williams & Wilkins, 2006:927–32.

Netter FH. Atlas of Human Anatomy, 4th ed. Philadelphia, PA: Saunders/Elsevier, 2006: plates 139–143.

Snell RS. Clinical Anatomy by Regions, 8th ed. Baltimore, MD: Lippincott Williams & Wilkins, 2008:689–90, 750–1.

A 12-year-old boy complains of difficulty hearing with his left ear for the past 2 weeks. He states that music and voices seem "far away." His medical problems include allergic rhinitis and asthma. On examination, he is without fever, but his left ear drum displays a yellowish discoloration. The left drum moves very little with a puff of air. The right tympanic membrane appears normal.

◆ **What is the most likely diagnosis?**

◆ **What is the clinical anatomy for this condition?**

ANSWERS TO CASE 47: MIDDLE EAR EFFUSION

Summary: A 12-year-old boy with allergic rhinitis and asthma has a 2-week history of difficulty hearing with his left ear. He is afebrile but has yellowish discoloration of his left tympanic membrane, which does not move well with insufflation.

◆ **Most likely diagnosis:** Middle ear effusion

◆ **Clinical anatomy of the condition:** Middle ear fluid impedes sound transmission by the middle ear ossicles

CLINICAL CORRELATION

Sound waves collected by the auricle and external acoustic meatus (canal) produce vibration of the tympanic membrane. These vibrations are transferred in turn to the ear ossicles, the malleus, incus, and stapes. Vibrations of the stapes produce movements of the endolymph within the cochlea, which are converted to the nervous impulse responsible for the sensation of hearing. Fluid within the middle ear cavity (effusion) diminishes the vibrations of the tympanic membrane and the ear ossicles. Effusions develop in the middle ear secondary to obstruction of the pharyngotympanic (auditory) tube, as with upper respiratory infections or allergic reactions. The insufflation of air through the otoscope in this patient does not induce the normal fluttering of the ear drum, further suggesting an effusion. An infectious process is unlikely in this case because of the absence of a fever or a red ear drum. Treatment of effusions include antihistamines, decongestants, and, in severe cases, surgical incision of the tympanic membrane for drainage (myringotomy) and insertion of drainage tubes.

APPROACH TO THE EAR

Objectives

1. Be able to describe the anatomy of the external acoustic meatus (canal).
2. Be able to describe the anatomy of the tympanic membrane and the three ear ossicles.
3. Be able to identify the structures of the middle ear cavity and those that communicate with it.

Definitions

Insufflation: Act of blowing a powder or gas into a body cavity, in this case through the otoscope, to assess whether there is fluid in the middle ear.

Perilymph/endolymph: The bony labyrinth of the inner ear contains the membranous labyrinth. Within the lumen of the membranous ducts is endolymph, a fluid similar in composition to intracellular fluid (low sodium, high potassium). The space between the ducts and the bony walls is filled with perilymph, a fluid similar in composition to normal extracellular fluid (high sodium, low potassium). The compartments that are filled with perilymph and endolymph do not communicate.

Effusion: Spread of a liquid into a space. In this case, the fluid is from the inflammatory response to the allergy.

Myringotomy: Procedure in which the tympanic membrane is pierced and tubes are inserted into the opening to drain the exudate.

DISCUSSION

The **external ear** is composed of the **auricle,** an elastic cartilage structure covered with skin and having several named parts, one of which is the **concha,** which funnels sound waves down the **external acoustic meatus or canal** (Figure 47-1). The **meatus** is lined with skin, and the wall of the lateral third is cartilaginous, whereas the medial two-thirds are bony. It has an anteromedial S-shaped course, which can be straightened by posterosuperior traction on the auricle.

The medial end of the meatus is closed by the tympanic membrane, a somewhat cone-shaped, 1-cm membrane composed of collagen and elastic fibers that is covered externally by thin skin and lined internally by the mucous membrane of the middle ear. The apex of the membrane's cone is called the **umbo.** The reflected light of an otoscope, the **cone of light,** originates at the umbo and is directed **anteroinferiorly.** A process of the **malleus,** called the handle, is applied to the medial surface of the membrane, and its tip is also attached at the umbo. The malleus has a lateral process that bulges the superior portion of

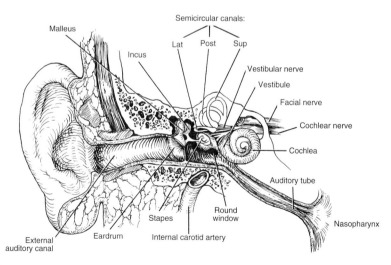

Figure 47-1. The middle ear. (*Reproduced, with permission, from Lindner HH. Clinical Anatomy. East Norwalk, CT: Appleton & Lange, 1989:76.*)

the membrane laterally. The portion superior to the lateral process is the **pars flaccida,** and the remainder of the membrane is called the **pars tensa.** The three ear ossicles are the **malleus, incus, and stapes,** lateral to medial, across the tympanic or middle ear cavity. Each bone has distinctive features. With a normal tympanic membrane, the handle of the malleus is clearly visible, and the long process of the incus is often visible posterior to the malleus. The **stapes** is shaped much like a **stirrup,** and its footplate fits into the oval window on the medial wall of the tympanic cavity. Its in-and-out movement transmits pressure waves through the **endolymph** within the **cochlea,** where the nerve impulses for hearing are generated. Excessive movements of the ear ossicles with loud noise are dampened by the tensor tympani muscle attached to the malleus and the stapedius muscle attached to the stapes. These **muscles are innervated by CN V and CN VII, respectively.**

The **tympanic cavity** is contained within the **petrous portion of the temporal bone.** Its features are usually described as being contained within a box with a roof, 4 walls, and a floor. Table 47-1 lists the bony features, related structures, and openings for each of the walls. The tympanic cavity is lined with a mucous membrane and contains the **chorda tympani branch of CN VII and the tympanic plexus (CN IX)** in addition to the ear ossicles and their associated muscles. Air pressure within the cavity is equalized with the nasopharynx through the pharyngotympanic or auditory tube.

Table 47-1
WALLS OF THE TYMPANIC CAVITY

	ROOF	FLOOR	LATERAL WALL	MEDIAL WALL	ANTERIOR WALL	POSTERIOR WALL
Bony feature	Tegmen tympani of temporal bone		Tympanic membrane, malleus, epitympanic recess	Promontory, prominence of facial canal, prominence of lateral semicircular canal		Mastoid process, pyramid
Related structure	Middle cranial fossa	Internal jugular vein	External acoustic meatus, chorda tympani	Vestibular apparatus, CN VII	Carotid artery, tensor tympani muscle	Mastoid air cells, CN VII, stapedius muscle
Opening					Auditory tube	Mastoid aditus

COMPREHENSION QUESTIONS

[47.1] A 4-year-old boy was noted to have recurrent ear infections. He underwent placement of tubes in the tympanic membranes 3 days previously
and currently complains of some difficulty in tasting candy. Which of
the following is the most likely explanation?

A. Disruption of CN VIII
B. Disruption of the chorda tympani
C. Effects of the anesthesia
D. Effects of the endotracheal tube

[47.2] A 5-year-old girl complains of severe pain from her right ear due to an
acute otitis media. Which of the following nerves is most likely responsible for carrying the sensation of pain from the tympanic membrane?

A. CN VII
B. CN VIII
C. CN IX
D. CN X

[47.3] A 3-year-old boy had three episodes of otitis media over the past year.
His mother asks the doctor why children tend to develop more ear
infections than adults. Which of the following is the most likely
anatomical explanation?

A. Changes in the eustachian tube
B. Changes in the external pinna
C. Changes in the external ear canal
D. Changes in the stapedius ossicle

Answers

[47.1]   **B.** The chorda tympani, which a branch of CN VII, courses behind
the tympanic membrane and occasionally can be injured during surgery for ear tubes. The chorda tympani innervates the anterior two-
thirds of the tongue.

[47.2]   **C.** The glossopharyngeal nerve (CN IX) is the afferent nerve for the
sensory input from the internal surface of the tympanic membrane
and the tympanic cavity.

[47.3]   **A.** The eustachian tube connects the middle ear to the oral cavity. The
eustachian tube is shorter and more horizontal in a child than in an
adult.

ANATOMY PEARLS

❖ The outer one-third of the external acoustic meatus is cartilaginous, thereby facilitating the straightening of its S-shaped curvature.
❖ The cone of light is seen in the anteroinferior quadrant of the tympanic membrane.
❖ The tensor tympani and stapedius muscles of the middle ear are innervated by CN V and CN VII, respectively.
❖ The tympanic cavity communicates with the nasopharynx through the pharyngotympanic (auditory) tube.

REFERENCES

Moore KL, Dalley AF. Clinically Oriented Anatomy, 5th ed. Baltimore, MD: Lippincott Williams & Wilkins, 2006:1022–36.
Netter FH. Atlas of Human Anatomy, 4th ed. Philadelphia, PA: Saunders/Elsevier, 2006: plates 93–4, 97–8.
Snell RS. Clinical Anatomy by Regions, 8th ed. Baltimore, MD: Lippincott Williams & Wilkins, 2008:706–15.

A 10-year-old girl is brought to her pediatrician's office complaining of headache for the past 2 weeks. Her mother had taken the girl to an optometrist, and her vision was normal. The patient states that she has been in good health and that she received a cat as a birthday present 1 month previously. On examination, she has a normal temperature, the tympanic membranes appear normal, and her throat is clear. There is some tenderness of the right cheek and over the right orbit.

◆ **What is the most likely diagnosis?**

◆ **What is the anatomical explanation for this condition?**

ANSWERS TO CASE 48: SINUSITIS

Summary: A 10-year-old girl who had recently acquired a cat has had a headache for a 2-week duration. She is afebrile, with normal-appearing tympanic membranes and throat. She has right maxillary and frontal tenderness.

◆ **Most likely diagnosis:** Maxillary and frontal sinusitis

◆ **Anatomical explanation for this condition:** Blocked drainage of the sinuses secondary to an allergic reaction of the nasal mucosa

CLINICAL CORRELATION

Sinusitis, a condition common in Americans, is an inflammation of one or more of the six sets of paranasal sinuses, most of which are related to the orbits. Inflammation may be caused by viruses, allergies, and bacterial pathogens. The sinuses are usually sterile cavities that are lined by ciliated mucosa rich in mucous cells, and mucus drains directly into the nasal cavities through small openings, or ostia. Edema of the nasal mucosa can easily occlude these openings and lead to secondary infection. The maxillary sinus is most commonly involved, and sinus pain or pressure sensation is typical. Transillumination of the sinuses that demonstrates opacification may be helpful on physical examination. Radiographs may also be helpful; CT imaging is usually reserved for complicated cases. The recent acquisition of a cat by the patient suggests maxillary and frontal sinusitis caused by an allergy rather than an infectious agent. Oral or topical (spray) decongestants, antihistamines, and/or nasal steroids are often helpful. Antibiotics are not indicated at this time, but the patient should be instructed to watch for development of fever or an increase in tenderness. Complications include osteomyelitis, ocular cellulitis, and cavernous sinus thrombophlebitis.

APPROACH TO THE SINUSES

Objectives

1. Be able to describe the location of the paranasal sinuses in the facial skeleton.
2. Be able to list the openings in the nasal cavity through which the paranasal sinuses drain.

Definitions

Osteomyelitis: Condition in which the bone and bone marrow become infected.

Thrombophlebitis: Condition in which a vein becomes inflamed in response to a blood clot.

DISCUSSION

The **paranasal sinuses are extensions of the nasal cavities into bones of the skull** and are **named for the bones in which they are located** (Figure 48-1). These spaces are lined with respiratory mucosa, decrease the weight of the skull, and probably assist in humidifying inspired air. See Case 51 for the anatomy of the nasal cavity. The **sphenoid sinuses** are located within the sphenoid bone, are variable in size and number, and open into the sphenoethmoidal recess. The **ethmoidal sinuses** consist of a series of sinuses positioned between the medial wall of the orbit and the nasal cavity (at the level of the bridge of the nose). For descriptive purposes, they are divided into anterior, middle, and posterior ethmoidal cells, and each has a separate opening. The **posterior ethmoidal cells have their opening in the superior nasal meatus.** The **middle ethmoidal cells** elevate the ethmoid bone in the middle meatus, thus creating the ethmoid bulla on whose surface these cells have their opening. Inferior to the ethmoid bulla is a groove, the semilunar hiatus. The **anterior ethmoidal cells** open into the anterior portion of the hiatus, called the **infundibulum.**

The **largest sinuses are the maxillary and frontal sinuses,** and their relatively large openings also drain into the **middle meatus.** The large **maxillary sinus** hollows the maxillary bone. The roof of the sinus, which also forms the floor of the orbit, is very thin and at risk in direct trauma to the orbit that causes sudden increases in pressure. Such trauma may cause **"blow-out" fractures** of the orbital floor. The opening of the maxillary sinus is found in the semilunar hiatus. The **frontal sinuses** are found in the frontal bone between the inner and outer tables and in the portion that forms the roof of the orbit. It is drained by the **frontonasal duct,** which opens into the infundibulum, the anterior portion of the semilunar hiatus.

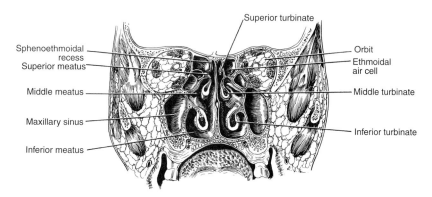

Figure 48-1. Sinuses in the coronal view. (*Reproduced, with permission, from Lindner HH. Clinical Anatomy. East Norwalk, CT: Appleton & Lange, 1989:68.*)

COMPREHENSION QUESTIONS

[48.1] A 24-year-old medical student has been diagnosed with sinusitis and asks her physician why there is nasal drainage during the night but not during the day. Which of the following is the best explanation?

A. Location of the ostia within the sinus
B. Location of the ostia within the nasal passage
C. Disruption of the drainage due to mastication
D. Diurnal mucus production increases at night

[48.2] A 22-year-old college student is being seen for possible sinusitis. The physician sees purulent drainage arising from the superior nasal meatus. Which of the following sinuses is likely to be infected?

A. Frontal
B. Maxillary
C. Sphenoidal
D. Ethmoidal

[48.3] A 28-year-old neuroanatomy graduate student noted pain at the bridge of his nose and had been told that he had "sinus" infections. He was speculating about the afferent nerve supply from this area. Which of the following is the most accurate description of the sensory nerve innervation?

A. Branches of CN III
B. Branches of CN V
C. Branches of CN VII
D. Branches of CN IX

Answers

[48.1]   **A.** The sinus most likely affected is the maxillary sinus. The ostia within the sinus are located superiorly in a location inefficient for gravity drainage. During sleep at night, the mucus flows out through the ostia.

[48.2]   **D.** The posterior ethmoidal sinus drains into the superior nasal meatus.

[48.3]   **B.** The paranasal sinuses are innervated by branches of CN V.

ANATOMY PEARLS

❖ The paranasal sinuses are named after the bones in which they are found (frontal, ethmoid, sphenoid, and maxilla).

❖ The maxillary, frontal, anterior, and posterior ethmoidal sinuses open into the middle nasal meatus.

❖ The maxillary sinus is the largest of the paranasal sinuses and is the most commonly infected sinus because its ostia are located superiorly.

❖ Trauma to the orbit may result in a blow-out fracture and, hence, orbital structures (such as extraocular muscles) may be pushed inferiorly into the maxillary sinus.

REFERENCES

Moore KL, Dalley AF. Clinically Oriented Anatomy, 5th ed. Baltimore, MD: Lippincott Williams & Wilkins, 2006:1016–22.

Netter FH. Atlas of Human Anatomy, 4th ed. Philadelphia, PA: Saunders/Elsevier, 2006: plates 48–50.

Snell RS. Clinical Anatomy by Regions, 8th ed. Baltimore, MD: Lippincott Williams & Wilkins, 2008:799–802.

A 7-year-old boy was referred to an ear-nose-throat (ENT) specialist after having recurrent episodes of tonsillitis with peritonsillar abscesses. His mother noted about seven infections over the past 8 months, all treated with antibiotics. After discussing treatment options with the family, the ENT recommended a tonsillectomy. The patient's tonsillectomy was complicated by bleeding from the surgical bed, and he had temporary loss of taste sensation from his posterior tongue. He is currently doing well and without complaints.

◆ **The intraoperative bleeding was most likely from which blood vessel?**

◆ **Why was there a temporary loss of taste sensation?**

ANSWERS TO CASE 49: RECURRENT TONSILLITIS

Summary: 7-year-old boy status post-tonsillectomy for recurrent tonsillitis complicated by increased intraoperative bleeding and temporary loss of taste sensation from the posterior one-third of the tongue.

◆ **Vessel involved with intraoperative bleeding:** External palatine vein

◆ **Loss of taste sensation:** Compression of glossopharyngeal nerve (CN IX)

CLINICAL CORRELATION

For patients with recurrent episodes of tonsillitis or peritonsillar abscesses (>4 episodes per year), tonsillectomy may be indicated. Although tonsillectomy is thought of as a routine procedure, it is not without its complications/risks. A thorough understanding of the anatomy of the pharynx is necessary in order to limit complications. The tonsillar bed is extremely vascular with the most common source of intraoperative bleeding from the external palatine vein which arises from the lateral aspect of the tonsillar bed. Even if a direct injury does not take place, compression from edema may cause temporary injury as in this case. Compression of glossopharyngeal nerve branches causes a temporary loss in taste sensation on the posterior aspect of the tongue. As the swelling goes down, so does the nerve impairment. Many other vital vessels, nerves, and structures are adjacent to the tonsils and care must be taken to avoid injury.

APPROACH TO THE TONSILS

Objectives

1. Be able to describe the divisions of the pharynx.
2. Be able to list the muscles that form the pharynx.
3. Be able to describe the components of the tonsillar ring.
4. Be able to identify vessels that supply the pharynx, especially branches that course through the tonsillar beds.
5. Be able to identify the cranial nerves providing sensory and motor innervation to the pharynx.

DISCUSSION

The **pharynx** is a space within the head that connects the **oral and nasal cavities** to the **trachea** and **esophagus**. Air-filled spaces in the temporal bone (i.e., the tympanic cavity and the mastoid air cells) connect with the pharynx through the **pharyngotympanic (Eustachian) tube.** The walls of the pharynx are covered with mucosa. Deep to the mucosa are several aggregations of lymphoid tissue that form a ring around the pharynx, priming the immune system for defense against pathogens (see Figure 49-1).

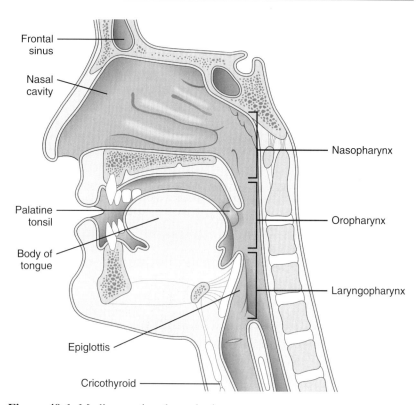

Frontal sinus

Nasal cavity

Palatine tonsil

Body of tongue

Epiglottis

Cricothyroid

Nasopharynx

Oropharynx

Laryngopharynx

Figure 49-1. Median section through pharynx.

The superior boundary of the pharynx is the base of the skull. The muscles of the pharyngeal walls form a cone that narrows to the esophagus. The medial pterygoid plates support the lateral walls of the superior part of the pharynx. The bodies of cervical vertebrae support the posterior wall. The anterior wall is interrupted by three apertures. One opens to the nasal cavity, another to the oral cavity, and a third to the larynx. Therefore, the pharynx is divided into three corresponding regions, the **nasopharynx, oropharynx,** and **laryngopharynx.** The naso- and oropharynx are continuous, but are separated by elevation of the soft palate during swallowing to prevent reflux of food and liquid into the nasopharynx. The oro- and laryngopharynx are also continuous. Depression of the **epiglottis** during swallowing separates the larynx from the laryngopharynx, preventing aspiration into the trachea and lungs.

The pharyngeal wall is composed of three muscles, the **superior, middle, and inferior pharyngeal constrictors.** The inferior part of the inferior constrictor muscle thickens as it merges with the esophagus, forming a sphincter called the **cricopharyngeus muscle.** The three constrictor muscles are stacked like ice-cream cones. Between the pairs of muscles are gaps that transmit important structures. The gap between the superior constrictor and the occipital bone transmits the pharyngotympanic tube, **levator veli palatini muscle**, and the **ascending palatine artery.** Between the superior and middle constrictors are the glossopharyngeal nerve and **stylopharyngeus muscle.** Between the middle and inferior constrictors course the **internal laryngeal nerve** and **superior laryngeal artery.** The **recurrent laryngeal nerve** and **inferior laryngeal artery** ascend deep to the inferior constrictor.

The lymphoid tissue surrounding the pharynx is commonly called the **Waldeyer ring,** which is composed of three masses of lymphoid tissue: the **pharyngeal tonsils** (also called **"adenoids"** when enlarged), the **palatine tonsils,** and the **lingual tonsils.** The pharyngeal tonsils are located in the roof and posterior wall of the nasopharynx. The opening of the pharyngotympanic tube into the nasopharynx is protected by a tonsil. The palatine tonsils are located in the anterior wall of the oropharynx between the **palatoglossal and palatopharyngeal folds**. The lingual tonsil is located under the mucosa of the posterior one-third of the tongue.

The pharynx is supplied by arteries from several sources, most of which are branches of the external carotid artery, specifically the **maxillary, facial, lingual, and superior thyroid arteries.** The constrictor muscles are also supplied by branches from the **deep cervical and the inferior thyroid arteries.** With respect to this case, the most important vessels are the ascending palatine and tonsillar branches of the facial artery. Surgery to remove the palatine tonsil can damage the tonsillar branch, resulting in excessive bleeding. Venous drainage from the pharynx parallels the arterial supply. In addition, there is an extensive **pharyngeal venous plexus** on the posterior surface of the constrictor muscles. The **external palatine vein** descends along the lateral surface of the palatine tonsil to drain into the venous plexus. Therefore, this vessel may be damaged during surgery to remove a palatine tonsil, also resulting in excessive bleeding.

The nerve supply to the pharynx is from cranial nerves IX and X. The **glossopharyngeal nerve (CN IX)** supplies general sensory fibers to the mucosa of the pharynx. These fibers contribute to the **afferent limb of the gag reflex.** CN IX also supplies special sensory fibers mediating taste to the posterior one-third of the tongue. This nerve exits the cranium through the **jugular foramen,** and descends with the **stylopharyngeus muscle** to pass through the gap between the superior and middle pharyngeal constrictor muscles. The vagus nerve (CN X) supplies general motor fibers to the constrictor muscles. These fibers contribute to the **efferent limb of the gag reflex.** This nerve also exits the cranium through the jugular foramen, but descends within the carotid sheath. As it descends, it gives off branches that form the pharyngeal plexus on the posterior surface of the pharynx. In this case, edema from the tonsillectomy compressed the branches of CN IX, blocking the sensation of taste from the posterior one-third of the tongue.

COMPREHENSION QUESTIONS

[49.1] During a procedure to remove a palatine tonsil, the operating field was suddenly filled with bright red blood. Which artery was inadvertently damaged?

A. Tonsillar branch of facial
B. Ascending pharyngeal
C. Ascending palatine
D. Descending palatine
E. Lingual

[49.2] A patient has a mild chronic cough, but has clear lungs and no evidence of bronchitis. Her physician believes that the symptoms are due to postnasal drip brought on by allergy. Which nerve is responsible for the afferent limb of the cough reflex?

A. CN V2
B. CN V3
C. CN VII
D. CN IX
E. CN X

[49.3] Which structure passes through the gap between the superior and middle constrictor muscles?

A. Recurrent laryngeal artery
B. Internal laryngeal nerve
C. Superior laryngeal artery
D. Glossopharyngeal nerve
E. Pharyngotympanic tube

Answers

[49.1] **A.** The tonsillar branch of the facial artery lies in the bed of the palatine tonsil and is susceptible to damage. Although the ascending palatine artery sends branches to the tonsil, it is not likely to be affected in a routine procedure.

[49.2] **D.** The cough reflex is stimulated by irritation of the laryngopharynx, which is innervated by CN IX. The trigeminal nerve (CN V1 and V2) innervates the oral and nasal cavities.

[49.3] **D.** The glossopharyngeal nerve (CN IX) passes through the gap between the superior and middle constrictors, along with the stylopharyngeus muscle and stylohyoid ligament.

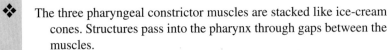

ANATOMY PEARLS

❖ The three pharyngeal constrictor muscles are stacked like ice-cream cones. Structures pass into the pharynx through gaps between the muscles.

❖ The tonsillar ring (Waldeyer) is a discontinuous mass of lymphoid tissue located where the body opens to the environment, exposing the immune system to pathogens.

❖ At the base of the palatine tonsil, the tonsillar branch of the facial artery, and the glossopharyngeal nerve (CN IX) can be identified.

❖ The gag reflex is evoked by mechanical stimulation of the oropharynx. The afferent limb of the reflex is mediated by the glossopharyngeal nerve (CN IX), and the efferent limb is mediated by the vagus nerve (CN X).

REFERENCES

Moore KL, Dalley AF. Clinically Oriented Anatomy, 5th ed. Baltimore, MD: Lippincott Williams & Wilkins, 2006:1101–10.

Netter FH. Atlas of Human Anatomy, 4th ed. Philadelphia, PA: Saunders/Elsevier, 2006: plates 63–4.

Snell RS. Clinical Anatomy by Regions, 8th ed. Baltimore, MD: Lippincott Williams & Wilkins, 2008:789–95.

A 47-year-old woman is undergoing surgical removal of her gallbladder (cholecystectomy). Her medical problems include insulin-dependent diabetes mellitus and sleep apnea. After the anesthesiologist has administered the paralyzing agent (succinylcholine), the patient is found to have spasms of the airway and difficulty breathing with the bag and mask. The anesthesiologist attempts to place an endotracheal tube by direct visualization (direct laryngoscopy), without success due to swelling (laryngeal edema). Meanwhile, the oxygen saturation content of the blood has decreased to a very low range of 80 percent. The anesthesiologist remarks that an emergency airway needs to be surgically opened.

◆ **What is your next step?**

◆ **What anatomical landmarks will be most helpful?**

ANSWERS TO CASE 50: EMERGENCY TRACHEOSTOMY

Summary: A 47-year-old woman who had diabetes and sleep apnea is undergoing elective cholecystectomy. After receiving the paralyzing agent, the patient develops laryngospasm and is difficult to ventilate. Direct laryngoscopy and intubation attempts are unsuccessful, and oxygen saturation is low.

◆ **Next step:** Emergency tracheostomy or cricothyroidotomy

◆ **Helpful anatomical landmarks:** Cricoid and thyroid laryngeal cartilages

CLINICAL CORRELATION

One of the leading causes of mortality at elective surgery is related to anesthesia, specifically an inability to ventilate the patient. This woman is probably obese and difficult to intubate due to a short neck, and her sleep apnea is a concern. When oxygen saturation decreases to dangerous levels (<90 percent), brain and/or heart ischemia may ensue. Immediate correction of oxygenation is critical, and, as in this case, emergency tracheostomy is indicated. One of the fastest methods is to enter the cricothyroid membrane in the midline, between the cricoid and thyroid laryngeal cartilages. This interval is usually palpable and is approximately one-third the distance from the top of the manubrium to the tip of the chin (mentum). A vertical incision is made in the membrane and a tracheal tube is inserted. Alternatively, a needle can be inserted into the same membrane, and oxygen administered through a jet ventilator. However, this procedure must be revised rapidly because there is insufficient flow to remove carbon dioxide from the lungs. Nonemergency tracheostomies are performed inferiorly to the cricoid cartilage and the isthmus of the thyroid gland.

APPROACH TO THE NECK UPPER AIRWAY

Objectives

1. Be able to list the landmarks of the anterior neck and identify the muscles of the infrahyoid region.
2. Be able to describe the cartilaginous skeleton of the larynx and the positions of the vocal cords in relation to palpable landmarks.
3. Be able to describe the thyroid gland's relationship to the larynx and its blood supply.

Definitions

ABCs: This mnemonic reminds us that the priorities of emergency management are airway, breathing, and circulation.

Endotracheal intubation: Placement of a tube through the mouth or nose and through the vocal cords to secure the airway and/or provide mechanical ventilation.

Tracheostomy: Surgical establishment of an airway by an opening from the skin to the trachea. These are emergent, when endotracheal intubation is impossible, or elective, when the patient has need of a long-term airway.

Cricothyroidotomy: Temporary method of establishing an airway by penetrating through the cricothyroid membrane. The procedure is nearly always performed emergently.

Cholecystectomy: Surgical procedure to remove the gallbladder.

Sleep apnea: Condition in which the patient in unable to breathe due to temporary obstruction of the airway, usually occurring during sleep. Loud snoring, choking, or periods of cessation of breathing are typical.

DISCUSSION

Deep to the thin skin of the anterior neck is the **platysma muscle,** which is within the **superficial fascia.** Deep to the platysma are the **infrahyoid (strap) muscles** of the neck. The paired **sternohyoid muscles** extend from the posterior surface of the manubrium to the hyoid bone, and their medial borders are just lateral and parallel to the midline. The superior bellies of the **omohyoid muscles** lie just lateral to the sternohyoid muscles. Deep to these muscles are found the **sternothyroid muscles** and continuing superiorly are the **thyrohyoid muscles.**

The skeleton of the **larynx** consists of the **U-shaped hyoid bone,** which lies at the level of the **C3 vertebra,** and nine cartilages. The **epiglottis, thyroid, and cricoid cartilages** are unpaired, whereas the **arytenoids, corniculate, and cuneiform are paired.** The thyroid cartilage, which resembles an open book, lies opposite the C4 and C5 vertebrae. Its two laminae are united anteriorly, and the **laryngeal prominence (Adam's apple)** is easily palpated and typically visible in men. The **cricoid cartilage is shaped like a signet ring,** with its larger laminar portion being posterior. It lies opposite the **C6 vertebra.** The thyroid cartilage is joined to the hyoid bone above and the cricoid cartilage below by ligaments and membranes. The **true vocal cords extend from the vocal processes of the arytenoid cartilages atop the lamina of the cricoid cartilage to the posterior surface of the thyroid cartilage superior to the lower border of the cartilage** (Figure 50-1). The interval between the thyroid and cricoid cartilages is closed by the cricothyroid membrane and is inferior to the true vocal cords (Figure 49-1). The cricothyroid muscle is also found laterally in this interval.

The **thyroid gland, like the larynx, is enclosed within the pretracheal fascia.** The large laterally placed lobes of the gland are applied to the surface of the laminae of the thyroid cartilage and the upper trachea, with the **parathyroid glands** embedded in their posterior surfaces. The right and left lobes are joined across the midline by the **isthmus,** which typically is inferior to the cricoid cartilage at the level of the second and third tracheal cartilage rings. In approximately 50 percent of individuals, a pyramidal lobe may be present that extends superiorly and overlies the cricothyroid membrane, but usually to one

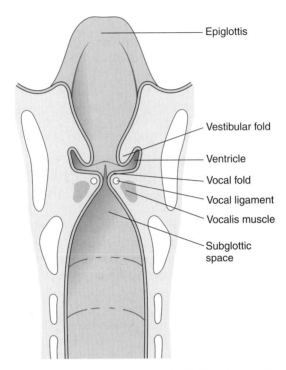

Figure 50-1. The larynx in coronal section including the vocal cords.

side of the midline. This **remnant of the thyroglossal duct** may be glandular or fibrous tissue. The thyroid and parathyroid glands are supplied by the paired **superior thyroid arteries** (direct branches from the **external carotid arteries**) and the **inferior thyroid arteries,** which are branches from the thyrocervical trunk. In 12 percent of individuals, a **small midline artery, the thyroid ima** artery, arises directly from the aortic arch or brachiocephalic trunk. It ascends on the anterior surface of the trachea to reach the isthmus.

COMPREHENSION QUESTIONS

[50.1] A 24-year-old man is being evaluated for airway abnormalities. Palpation of the cricoid cartilage is normally at which vertebral level?

A. C2

B. C4

C. C6

D. T1

[50.2] A 45-year-old woman is undergoing thyroid surgery for suspected thyroid cancer. The surgeon has taken a midline approach and encounters significant bleeding below the isthmus of the thyroid gland. Which of the following is the likely cause of the bleeding?

A. Penetration into the trachea
B. Superior thyroid artery
C. Inferior thyroid artery
D. Thyroid ima artery
E. Inferior laryngeal artery

[50.3] A 54-year-old woman has undergone partial thyroid resection due to a nontender cold nodule that likely represents cancer. One week after surgery, she complains of twitching of the right arm and "spasms" of both hands. Which of the following is the most likely explanation?

A. Anxiety after surgery
B. Effects of anesthesia
C. Parathyroid glands removed
D. Vagal nerve injury

[50.4] An emergency cricothyroidotomy is thought to be warranted due to airway collapse and severe laryngoedema. Which of the following is the most accurate description of the location of the cricothyroid membrane?

A. Immediately superior to the thyroid cartilage
B. Immediately inferior to the thyroid cartilage
C. Immediately inferior to the cricoid cartilage
D. Just deep to the isthmus of the thyroid gland
E. Immediately inferior to the hyoid bone

Answers

[50.1] **C.** The cricoid cartilage is usually located at the C6 vertebral level.

[50.2] **D.** In up to 12 percent of individuals, a small midline artery, called the thyroid ima artery, arises from the aortic arch or brachiocephalic trunk and reaches the thyroid isthmus inferiorly.

[50.3] **C.** The parathyroid glands are variably inside the thyroid gland. With resections of the thyroid, the small parathyroid glands may be affected, leading to decreased levels of calcitonin and, hence, hypocalcemia. The low calcium levels may cause clinical symptoms of muscle spasms, tetany, or even convulsions.

[50.4] **B.** The cricothyroid membrane is just inferior to the thyroid cartilage and superior to the cricoid cartilage.

ANATOMY PEARLS

❖ The cricoid cartilage lies at the level of the C6 vertebra.
❖ The true vocal cords lie superior to the cricothyroid membrane.
❖ The cricothyroid membrane is located inferior to the thyroid cartilage and superior to the cricoid cartilage.
❖ A pyramidal thyroid lobe may overlay the cricothyroid membrane close to the midline.
❖ In a small percentage of patients, a small midline artery, the thyroid ima, may directly supply the isthmus.

REFERENCES

Moore KL, Dalley AF. Clinically Oriented Anatomy, 5th ed. Baltimore, MD: Lippincott Williams & Wilkins, 2006:1083-1101.

Netter FH. Atlas of Human Anatomy, 4th ed. Philadelphia, PA: Saunders/Elsevier, 2006: plates 74, 77–8.

Snell RS. Clinical Anatomy by Regions, 8th ed. Baltimore, MD: Lippincott Williams & Wilkins, 2008:810–14, 817–8.

A 22-year-old male presents to the emergency department complaining of severe nasal bleeding for the past 30 minutes that he cannot stop. He denies any trauma, bleeding disorders, or use of medications such as aspirin or ibuprofen. The patient indicates that this nose bleed is unique because he is bleeding from both nostrils and blood is draining into his throat and choking him. He feels as though the blood were collecting in the back of his throat. He has tried "pinching" his nose, but the bleeding continues.

◆ **What is the most likely anatomical explanation for this condition?**

ANSWER TO CASE 51: EPISTAXIS

Summary: A 22-year-old male has had a 30-minute bilateral epistaxis with drainage of blood to the nasopharynx and choking. He denies trauma, bleeding disorders, or use of anticoagulant medications. Anterior nasal pinching did not help.

◆   **Most likely anatomical explanation:** Posterior epistaxis

CLINICAL CORRELATION

Epistaxis, or bleeding from the nose, is a common condition. Most cases arise from the anterior region of the nasal septum, and the bleeding site is fairly easy to visualize. Most anterior nose bleeds will respond to direct pressure, although other measures may be necessary, including topical vasoconstrictors such as cocaine, cautery, or nasal packing. This patient's epistaxis is atypical in that it is bilateral, with posterior drainage that produces a choking sensation. These symptoms suggest a posterior source, which is more difficult to control. Treatment of this type is by posterior nasal pack or a balloon tamponade device. Antibiotics are usually required to prevent sinusitis or toxic shock syndrome. Persistent or atypical epistaxis should alert the clinician to bleeding abnormalities. Patients who have congenital conditions such as hemophilia or von Willebrand disease may develop epistaxis. Acquired processes, such as use of aspirin or nonsteroidal anti-inflammatory medication, or frank anticoagulation with heparin or warfarin sodium (Coumadin) may be causative. Disease processes such as hepatic failure may lead to decreased levels of vitamin K–dependent coagulation factors.

APPROACH TO THE NOSE

Objectives

1.   Be able to list the features of the external nose and nasal cavity.
2.   Be able to describe the arterial supply to the nasal cavities.

Definitions

Epistaxis: Bleeding from the nose, usually divided clinically into an anterior or a posterior source.

Kiesselbach plexus: Area on the anterior portion of the nasal septum that is very vascular because of the anastomosis of blood vessels; this is the most common site for epistaxis.

Coagulopathy: Abnormalities to the normal pathways of hemostasis that lead to bleeding. Causes are usually congenital or acquired.

Anticoagulant: Chemical that interferes with the normal process of blood clotting.

DISCUSSION

The **external nose** is composed of the paired nasal bones, which form the bridge of the nose, and adjacent portions of the frontal bones and maxillae. The majority of the external nose is **cartilaginous** and is formed by the paired **alar** and **lateral nasal cartilages** and the **unpaired septal cartilage.** The anterior opening into the nasal cavity is the anterior nares. The nasal cavity is a somewhat pyramidal space within the skull between the two orbits. It is subdivided into right and left nasal cavities by the **nasal septum,** which is formed by the **vomer bone, perpendicular plate** of the **ethmoid bone,** nasal crests of the maxilla and palatine bones, and the **septal cartilage.** The roof of each cavity is formed by the **frontal, ethmoid, and sphenoid bones,** and its floor is formed by the palatine portion of the maxilla and the **horizontal plate of the palatine bone.** The posterior openings of each nasal cavity into the nasopharynx are the posterior **choanae.**

The complex lateral walls are formed by portions of the nasal, maxilla, ethmoid, and palatine bones. The surface area of the lateral walls is increased by the three nasal **conchae.** The **superior and middle conchae** are features of the **ethmoid bone,** whereas the **inferior nasal concha is an individual bone.** The posterosuperior portion of the nasal cavity, superior to the superior conchae, is the **sphenoethmoid recess.** Inferior to each of the conchae is a space named for the concha immediately superior to it. Thus, the superior, middle, and inferior nasal meatuses lie inferiorly to the superior, middle, and inferior nasal conchae, respectively. Each nasal cavity is lined with a highly vascular mucosa whose function is to warm and humidify inspired air (Figure 51-1).

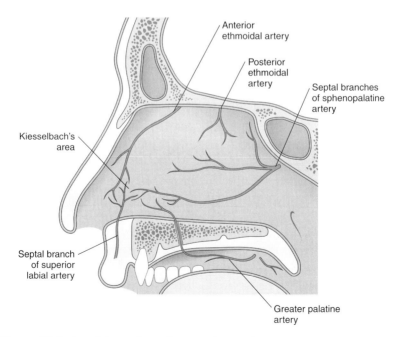

Figure 51-1. Arterial supply to the nose (septum).

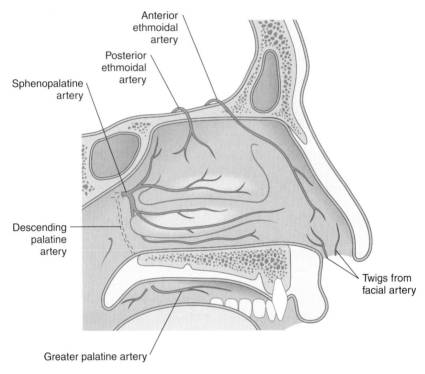

Figure 51-2. Arterial supply to the nose (lateral wall).

Each nasal cavity is supplied by nasal branches of the **sphenopalatine artery, anterior and posterior ethmoidal arteries, greater palatine artery, and superior labial and lateral nasal branches of the facial artery** (Figure 51-2). These arteries anastomose at **Kiesselbach area** on the anterior portion of the nasal septum (opposite the anterior end of the inferior concha). This is the **most common site for epistaxis.**

COMPREHENSION QUESTIONS

[51.1] A 55-year-old man has become anemic and hypotensive due to severe anterior epistaxis. An ear-nose-throat surgeon has been called to address the bleeding. He states that he may need to occlude the major arterial supply. Which of the following arteries is most likely to be responsible?

   A. Ethmoidal
   B. Sphenopalatine
   C. Superior labial
   D. Greater palatine

[51.2] An 18-year-old woman arrives in the emergency department complaining of persistent epistaxis. On examination, there is bleeding from the right nostril. Which of the following locations is the most likely source of the bleeding?

A. Anterior nasal septum
B. Posterior nasal septum
C. Anterior turbinate
D. Posterior turbinate
E. Nasal floor

[51.3] An 18-year-old woman is thrown from her car during a motor vehicle accident and hits her head against the pavement. She has lost consciousness but currently is alert and has equally reactive pupils. She is well except for clear nasal leakage from the right nostril that has not abated over 24 hours. Which of the following is the most likely etiology?

A. Sympathetic sinus drainage
B. Allergic rhinitis from the air bag
C. Damage to the cribriform plate
D. Lacrimonasal fistula

Answers

[51.1] **B.** The major blood supply to the anterior septum is the sphenopalatine artery, a branch of which supplies the nasal septum. The sphenopalatine artery arises from the maxillary artery, which is a terminal branch of the external carotid artery.

[51.2] **A.** The most common location of epistaxis is the region of the anterior septum known as Kiesselbach plexus, which has a rich anastomosis of arteries.

[51.3] **C.** This patient likely has cerebrospinal fluid (CSF) rhinorrhea, which is not unusual after head trauma. The cribriform plate and meninges are disrupted, which allows CSF to leak through the nose. This predisposes to meningitis.

ANATOMY PEARLS

❖ The anterior portion of the nasal septum is cartilaginous.
❖ The superior and middle nasal conchae are features of the ethmoid bone.
❖ The most common site for epistaxis is where the several arteries that supply the nasal cavity anastomose on the anterior nasal septum (Kiesselbach area).

REFERENCES

Moore KL, Dalley AF. Clinically Oriented Anatomy, 5th ed. Baltimore, MD: Lippincott Williams & Wilkins, 2006:1013–9.

Netter FH. Atlas of Human Anatomy, 4th ed. Philadelphia, PA: Saunders/Elsevier, 2006: plates 37–41.

Snell RS. Clinical Anatomy by Regions, 8th ed. Baltimore, MD: Lippincott Williams & Wilkins, 2008:795–800.

A 45-year-old woman complains of a left posterior toothache for the past 2 weeks that she treated with salt water gargles. However, over the past 24 hours, she has had fever and difficulty opening her mouth while talking or swallowing. On examination, the patient has a fever of 101°F, with redness of the left submandibular region extending to the left side of her throat. She is sitting up but anxious and drooling and has some inspiratory stridor. The physician states that the infection in the mouth has spread to the neck and may finally enter into the chest.

◆ **What is the most likely diagnosis?**

◆ **What is the anatomical mechanism for this condition?**

ANSWERS TO CASE 52: DENTAL ABSCESS/LUDWIG ANGINA

Summary: A 45-year-old woman had a left molar toothache for 2 weeks but now has fever, trismus, and dysphagia. There is a left submandibular inflammation extending to the left side of the throat. She is sitting but is anxious and drooling and has some inspiratory stridor. This infection may track from the mouth to the neck to the chest.

◆ **Most likely diagnosis:** Submandibular cellulitis (Ludwig angina)

◆ **Anatomical mechanism for this condition:** A dental (molar) abscess has tracked inferiorly from the submandibular space to impinge on the trachea

CLINICAL CORRELATION

Dental abscesses are relatively common occurrences and typically are self-limited or easily treated with antibiotics such as penicillin. Occasionally, an infection involving the molar teeth may extend into the submandibular space (Ludwig angina) and affect the trachea or carotid sheath contents. Fever, painful edema, limited neck mobility, drooling, and difficulty opening the mouth are clinical findings. The infection can also extend inferiorly into the mediastinum (mediastinitis). The inspiratory stridor in this case may indicate tracheal compression. In such cases, laryngoscopy may lead to laryngospasm and complete airway obstruction. Lateral neck radiographs or CT imaging are helpful in the diagnosis. The best treatment is intravenous antibiotics, airway protection (intubation if needed), and operative drainage of the abscess.

APPROACH TO THE ORAL CAVITY

Objectives

1. Be able to list the layers of the deep cervical fascia.
2. Be able to describe the structures in the floor of the mouth and sub-mandibular space and its communications with the spaces of the neck.
3. Be able to describe the route of spread of infection from the oral cavity into the thorax.

Definitions

Stridor: A high-pitched whispering sound with respiration that indicates obstruction of the airway.
Trismus: Sustained contraction of the masseter muscle, leading to "lockjaw."
Dysphagia: Difficulty or pain with swallowing.
Ligamentum nuchae: A thickened extension of the supraspinal ligament into the neck.

DISCUSSION

The **deep cervical fascia** consists of connective tissue sheets that enclose and support a variety of structures in the neck. Deep to the superficial fascia and **platysma,** the investing fascia (the superficial layer of deep fascia) **encircles the neck** and splits to enclose the **SCM** and the **trapezius muscles** and attach to the **ligamentum nuchae** posteriorly. Superiorly, it attaches to the **hyoid bone, mandible, and base of the skull;** inferiorly, it attaches to the **acromion, clavicle, and manubrium of the sternum.** The **prevertebral fascia** surrounds the cervical vertebral column, the spinal cord, and the pre- and paravertebral musculatures. It attaches to the base of the skull superiorly, the ligamentum nuchae posteriorly, and blends with the anterior longitudinal ligament of the vertebral column in the thorax. The **pretracheal fascia** surrounds the larynx, trachea, esophagus, thyroid, and parathyroid glands and splits to enclose the **infrahyoid (strap) muscles** of the neck. It is attached superiorly to the hyoid bone and inferiorly blends with the fibrous pericardium in the thorax. Posteriorly and superiorly, it is continuous with the **buccopharyngeal fascia.** The carotid **sheath** is usually described as being formed from the investing, prevertebral and pretracheal layers.

Between the prevertebral and buccopharyngeal fascias lies the **retropharyngeal space** ("danger space"). This space is a pathway for spread of infection to the thorax, possibly resulting in cardiac tamponade. Within the pretracheal fascia is a potential space filled with loose areolar connective tissue called the visceral space (Figure 52-1).

The **submandibular space** lies between the mucosa of the floor of the mouth and the mylohyoid and hyoglossus muscles. The root of the tongue lies medially, and the inner surface of the mandible lies laterally. The space contains the **sublingual gland and ducts,** a portion of the submandibular gland and its duct, and the lingual and hypoglossal nerves. A cleft exists between the mylohyoid and hyoglossus muscles, through which the submandibular gland wraps around the posterior border of the mylohyoid muscle. The roots of the **posterior molar teeth** are close to the inner surface of the mandible, thus increasing the risk of dental abscesses **spreading into the submandibular space. Infectious material can thus spread inferiorly into the visceral space through the cleft between the mylohyoid and hyoglossus muscles.**

Figure 52-1. Compartments of the neck: 1 = investing fascia, 2 = sternoclei-domastoid muscle, 3 = infrahyoid muscle, 4 = trapezius muscle, 5 = visceral (pretracheal) fascia, 6 = thyroid gland, 7 = trachea, 8 = recurrent laryngeal nerve, 9 = esophagus, 10 = buccopharyngeal fascia, 11 = alar fascia (present only in upper pharynx), 12 = retropharyngeal (retroesophageal) space, 13 = neurovascular (carotid) sheath, 14 = common carotid artery, 15 = internal jugular vein, 16 = vagus nerve, 17 = prevertebral fascia, 18 = phrenic nerve, 19 = sympathetic trunk, 20 = roots of the brachial plexus, 21 = vertebral artery. (*Reproduced, with permission, from the University of Texas Health Science Center, Houston Medical School.*)

COMPREHENSION QUESTIONS

[52.1] A 67-year-old man developed a dental abscess that he ignored for 2 weeks. At that time, he began to have severe chest pain due to infection of the mediastinum. Through which pathway did the infection most likely spread to the mediastinum?

A. Masticator space
B. Pretracheal space
C. Retropharyngeal space
D. Suprasternal space

[52.2] A dentist uses local anesthesia to prepare for a procedure on a lower molar tooth. Which of the following nerves is the dentist blocking?

A. Submental
B. Maxillary
C. Mandibular
D. Vagus

[52.3] A 24-year-old male was involved in a knife fight in a bar. He appeared in the emergency department with a 2-cm laceration in the anterolateral neck. The wound was superficial, but the physician observed muscle fibers just deep to the superficial fascia. Which of the following muscles was observed?

A. Platysma
B. Sternocleidomastoid
C. Omohyoid
D. Trapezius
E. Thyrohyoid

Answers

[52.1] **C.** The major pathway between the infections of the neck and the chest is through the retropharyngeal space, which is a potential space between the prevertebral layer of fascia and the buccopharyngeal fascia surrounding the pharynx.

[52.2] **C.** Dental anesthesia involving the lower molar teeth is called a lower mandibular block. The nerve affected is the inferior alveolar nerve branch of the mandibular nerve, which is a branch of V3.

[52.3] **A.** The platysma muscle is a wide flat muscle that covers the anterolateral region of the neck.

ANATOMY PEARLS

 The submandibular space is continuous with the visceral space in the neck.

 The investing, pretracheal, and prevertebral deep cervical fascias contribute to the carotid sheath.

 The major pathway for infection between the neck and the chest is the retropharyngeal space.

REFERENCES

Moore KL, Dalley AF. Clinically Oriented Anatomy, 5th ed. Baltimore, MD: Lippincott Williams & Wilkins, 2006:1049–53.

Netter FH. Atlas of Human Anatomy, 4th ed. Philadelphia, PA: Saunders/Elsevier, 2006: plates 35, 67, 73.

Snell RS. Clinical Anatomy by Regions, 8th ed. Baltimore, MD: Lippincott Williams & Wilkins, 2008:743–7.

A 3-day-old female infant is noted to have excessive tearing of the left eye and a small, firm, pea-size mass at the inferior region of the junction between the eye and the nose (oculonasal junction). The mass is not inflamed, and the infant is otherwise in good health and feeding well.

◆ **What is the most likely diagnosis?**

◆ **What is the anatomical explanation for this disorder?**

ANSWERS TO CASE 53: LACRIMAL SAC ENLARGEMENT

Summary: A 3-day-old healthy infant has excessive tearing of the left eye and a small, firm, pea-size mass inferior to the medial canthus.

◆   **Most likely diagnosis:** Lacrimal sac enlargement (dacryocystocele)

◆   **Anatomical explanation of the disorder:** Congenital atresia of ducts draining into or out of the lacrimal sac

CLINICAL CORRELATION

The tear drainage system begins at the lacrimal puncta at the medial portion between the upper and lower eyelids. The puncta open into lacrimal canaliculi, which terminate at the lacrimal sac, and in turn are drained by the nasolacrimal duct. The nasolacrimal duct develops from a solid cord of cells that recanalizes to establish the lumen of the duct and terminates in the inferior nasal meatus. Atresia of the duct (due to failure to recanalize) occurs in 1 to 3 percent of newborns. Atresia of the lacrimal canaliculi presents with excessive tearing and without a mass. Nasolacrimal duct atresia presents as a mass due to enlargement of the lacrimal sac, and the mass accompanied by excessive tearing suggests atresia of the canaliculi and the nasolacrimal duct. Massage of the nasolacrimal duct region with watchful waiting is the usual treatment, and most cases resolve by age 6 months. Persistent obstruction after age 9 months warrants intervention, such as nasolacrimal duct probing. Care must be exercised to avoid creating a false tract. Because the canaliculi and duct are obstructed in this case, duct probing is indicated.

APPROACH TO THE LACRIMAL GLAND

Objectives

1. Be able to describe the anatomy of the lacrimal gland.
2. Be able to describe the pathway for drainage of tears from the ocular globe to the nasal cavity.

Definitions

Lacrimal duct probing: Outpatient surgical procedure whereby a thin metal probe is used to cannulate the lacrimal duct, which is presumably occluded.

Dacryocystocele: Enlargement of the lacrimal sac.

Canthus: Angle formed by the upper and lower eyelids.

Atresia: Absence of a normal opening due to a developmental defect.

DISCUSSION

The **lacrimal gland** is located in a shallow fossa at the superolateral aspect of the orbit (Figure 53-1). Approximately 12 small lacrimal ducts drain each gland, whose secretions or tears enter the **conjunctival sac superolaterally** at the superior conjunctival fornix, and wash over the surface of the eye in an inferomedial direction, aided by the blinking action of the eyelids. The lacrimal gland is innervated by **autonomic nerves,** with the secretomotor fibers being a part of **CN VII,** whereas the sympathetic fibers are vasoconstrictive. Both types of fibers reach the gland through the lacrimal branch of the ophthalmic division of CN V.

Tears accumulate at the medial angle of the eye in the lacrimal lake. At the medial ends of the upper and lower eyelids, a small elevation, the **lacrimal papilla,** has an opening or **puncta** that leads to the **lacrimal canaliculus.** The two canaliculi terminate in the **lacrimal sac,** a blind-ended membranous structure continuous inferiorly with the **nasolacrimal duct.** The duct passes through the nasolacrimal canal of each maxilla and terminates in the **inferior nasal meatus,** the space bounded by the inferior nasal concha. Tears then pass to the nasopharynx and are swallowed.

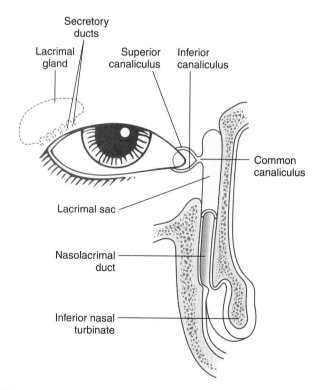

Figure 53-1. Lacrimal drainage system.

COMPREHENSION QUESTIONS

[53.1] A 30-year-old woman underwent blunt trauma to the left eye and found out that she was unable to secrete tears from that eye. Which of the following is the most likely location of the injury?

    A. Medial superior orbit
    B. Medial inferior orbit
    C. Lateral superior orbit
    D. Lateral inferior orbit
    E. Adjacent to nasal bridge

[53.2] A clinician places blue dye into the right eye to assess the patency of the tear duct system. Where should one look to see the eventual flow of the dye, assuming the lacrimal duct system is patent?

    A. Superior nasal meatus
    B. Middle nasal meatus
    C. Inferior nasal meatus
    D. Oral cavity
    E. Subclavian vein

[53.3] A 5-year-old boy is noted to have severe pain, swelling, and redness around his right eye. He has been diagnosed with periorbital cellulitis, with probable spread of the infection to the brain. Which of the following routes best describes the probable avenue of spread to the brain?

    A. Through the cribriform plate into the meningeal space
    B. Facial vein to ophthalmic vein to cavernous sinus into the dura space
    C. Frontal sinus into the sagittal sinus and into the subarachnoid space
    D. Facial canal through the internal auditory meatus to the posterior cranial fossa

Answers

[53.1] **C.** The lacrimal gland, which produces tears, is located in the superior and lateral aspects of the orbit.

[53.2] **C.** The tears flow through the puncta in the medial inferior aspect of the eyelid and travel through the lacrimal duct into the inferior nasal meatus.

[53.3] **B.** Infections involving the periorbital space can penetrate through the ophthalmic vein into the cavernous sinus and into the dural space, leading to meningitis. Thus, prompt antibiotic therapy is critical with this infection.

ANATOMY PEARLS

 The lacrimal gland is located at the superolateral portion of the orbit.
 The parasympathetic secretomotor fibers originate in CN VII.
Tears are produced by the lacrimal gland and drain through the lacrimal puncta into the lacrimal sac and through the nasolacrimal duct.
 The nasolacrimal duct terminates in the inferior nasal meatus.
 The most common cause of excessive tearing in a newborn is underdevelopment of the lacrimal duct, which is usually treated with expectant management.

REFERENCES

Moore KL, Dalley AF. Clinically Oriented Anatomy, 5th ed. Baltimore, MD: Lippincott Williams & Wilkins, 2006:961–4.

Netter FH. Atlas of Human Anatomy, 4th ed. Philadelphia, PA: Saunders/Elsevier, 2006: plates 81–2.

Snell RS. Clinical Anatomy by Regions, 8th ed. Baltimore, MD: Lippincott Williams & Wilkins, 2008:692–4.

Listing of Cases

Listing by Case Number

Listing by Disorder (Alphabetical)

LISTING BY CASE NUMBER

LISTING BY DISORDER (ALPHABETICAL)

❖ INDEX

Note: Page numbers followed by *f* or *t* indicate figures or tables, respectively.